DEADLY DISEASES AND EPIDEMICS

HIV/AIDS

DEADLY DISEASES AND EPIDEMICS

HIV/AIDS

Consuelo M. Beck-Sagué,
M.D., F.A.A.P.

Caridad C. Beck

CONSULTING EDITOR
The Late **I. Edward Alcamo**
Distinguished Teaching Professor of Microbiology,
SUNY Farmingdale

FOREWORD BY
David Heymann
World Health Organization

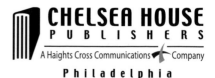

CHELSEA HOUSE
P U B L I S H E R S
A Haights Cross Communications Company
P h i l a d e l p h i a

Writing performed by Consuelo M. Beck-Sagué in her private capacity. No official support or endorsement by CDC is intended or should be inferred.

Dedication

We dedicate the books in the DEADLY DISEASES AND EPIDEMICS series to Ed Alcamo, whose wit, charm, intelligence, and commitment to biology education were second to none.

CHELSEA HOUSE PUBLISHERS

VP, NEW PRODUCT DEVELOPMENT Sally Cheney
DIRECTOR OF PRODUCTION Kim Shinners
CREATIVE MANAGER Takeshi Takahashi
MANUFACTURING MANAGER Diann Grasse

Staff for HIV and AIDS

ASSOCIATE EDITOR Beth Reger
PRODUCTION EDITOR Megan Emery
PHOTO EDITOR Sarah Bloom
SERIES DESIGNER Terry Mallon
COVER DESIGNER Keith Trego
LAYOUT 21st Century Publishing and Communications, Inc.

A Haights Cross Communications ✦ Company

http://www.chelseahouse.com

First Printing

1 3 5 7 9 8 6 4 2

Library of Congress Cataloging-in-Publication Data

Beck-Sague, Consuelo M., 1952–
    HIV and AIDS / Consuelo M. Beck-Sague, Caridad Beck.
       p. cm.—(Deadly diseases and epidemics)
Includes bibliographical references and index.
    ISBN 0-7910-7717-9 (hardcover)
    1. AIDS (Disease) I. Beck, Caridad, 1983– II. Title. III. Series.
RC606.6.B43 2003
616.97'92—dc22

                                                    2004001603

Table of Contents

Foreword

In the 1960s, many of the infectious diseases that had terrorized generations were tamed. After a century of advances, the leading killers of Americans both young and old were being prevented with new vaccines or cured with new medicines. The risk of death from pneumonia, tuberculosis (TB), meningitis, influenza, whooping cough, and diphtheria declined dramatically. New vaccines lifted the fear that summer would bring polio, and a global campaign was on the verge of eradicating smallpox worldwide. New pesticides like DDT cleared mosquitoes from homes and fields, thus reducing the incidence of malaria, which was present in the southern United States and which remains a leading killer of children worldwide. New technologies produced safe drinking water and removed the risk of cholera and other water-borne diseases. Science seemed unstoppable. Disease seemed destined to all but disappear.

But the euphoria of the 1960s has evaporated.

The microbes fought back. Those causing diseases like TB and malaria evolved resistance to cheap and effective drugs. The mosquito developed the ability to defuse pesticides. New diseases emerged, including AIDS, Legionnaires, and Lyme disease. And diseases which had not been seen in decades re-emerged, as the hantavirus did in the Navajo Nation in 1993. Technology itself actually created new health risks. The global transportation network, for example, meant that diseases like West Nile virus could spread beyond isolated regions and quickly become global threats. Even modern public health protections sometimes failed, as they did in 1993 in Milwaukee, Wisconsin, resulting in 400,000 cases of the digestive system illness cryptosporidiosis. And, more recently, the threat from smallpox, a disease believed to be completely eradicated, has returned along with other potential bioterrorism weapons such as anthrax.

The lesson is that the fight against infectious diseases will never end.

In our constant struggle against disease, we as individuals have a weapon that does not require vaccines or drugs, and that is the warehouse of knowledge. We learn from the history of science that "modern" beliefs can be wrong. In this series of books, for example, you will learn that diseases like syphilis were once thought to be caused by eating potatoes. The invention of the microscope set science on the right path. There are more positive lessons from history. For example, smallpox was eliminated by vaccinating everyone who had come in contact with an infected person. This "ring" approach to smallpox control is still the preferred method for confronting an outbreak, should the disease be intentionally reintroduced.

At the same time, we are constantly adding new drugs, new vaccines, and new information to the warehouse. Recently, the entire human genome was decoded. So too was the genome of the parasite that causes malaria. Perhaps by looking at the microbe and the victim through the lens of genetics we will to be able to discover new ways to fight malaria, which remains the leading killer of children in many countries.

Because of advances in our understanding of such diseases as AIDS, entire new classes of anti-retroviral drugs have been developed. But resistance to all these drugs has already been detected, so we know that AIDS drug development must continue.

Education, experimentation, and the discoveries that grow out of them are the best tools to protect health. Opening this book may put you on the path of discovery. I hope so, because new vaccines, new antibiotics, new technologies, and, most importantly, new scientists are needed now more than ever if we are to remain on the winning side of this struggle against microbes.

David Heymann
Executive Director
Communicable Diseases Section
World Health Organization
Geneva, Switzerland

Preface

No hay mal de que un bien no venga.

Dicho Cubano

("There is no evil from which some good does not come."

Cuban Saying)

We dedicate this book to all the children, women, and men worldwide living with HIV and to those whose compassionate care and brilliant research are making all the difference. In particular we dedicate this book to Ronald Valdiserri, M.D., M.P.H., and to our father and grandfather, Dr. Miguel Angel Sagué, who is so supportive of our work.

CBS, CCB

In June 1981, after completing my medical residency in pediatrics, I was about to start a job as a pediatrician in a clinic in Chicago. I dreaded leaving the Northeast and being far from my best friend from medical school in Philadelphia, Pennsylvania, Dr. Edwin (Eddie) Valdiserri, a brilliant, funny, kind, and caring person.

Before I moved to Chicago, I visited Eddie in Philadelphia. During that visit, Eddie and I discussed a recent article that had appeared in the *Morbidity and Mortality Weekly Report* (*MMWR*), a weekly newsletter published by the Centers for Disease Control and Prevention (CDC). The article was about five young, previously healthy homosexual men who had been treated for *Pneumocystis carinii* pneumonia and candida (yeast) infection of the mouth (thrush). Although these diseases were well known, they were never seen in healthy adults; these illnesses were seen only in people who had been treated with medicines that suppressed their immune defenses so they would not reject transplanted organs, or in other very severely ill patients.

The article stated that two of the men had died. Descriptions of the five patients' cases were very strange. These patients had never been seriously ill before. They had not had transplants. They had never taken medicines that could suppress their immune defenses.

They were healthy young adults. An editorial in the case reports included this sentence: "The fact that these patients were all homosexuals suggests an association between some aspect of a homosexual lifestyle or disease acquired through sexual contact and *Pneumocystis carinii* pneumonia in this population."[1] The article also stated that, "Two of the 5 reported having frequent homosexual contacts with various partners."

During the 1970s, many people, both homosexuals and heterosexuals, had sex with various partners. Rates of sexually transmitted diseases, infectious diseases spread during sexual intercourse, such as syphilis and gonorrhea, soared. The number of syphilis and rectal gonorrhea cases was particulary high among homosexual men.

After reading that article, we had no idea that a new disease had emerged. In medical school, we were taught that infectious diseases were declining in importance. In fact, one deadly infectious disease, smallpox, which had been a scourge for centuries, was completely eliminated while Eddie and I attended medical school in Philadelphia. The first time I realized that new infectious diseases could emerge was in 1976, when a new infectious disease, Legionnaires' disease, killed several people who had attended an American Legion meeting in Philadelphia. We were stunned to think that an epidemic of a new infectious disease could occur in the United States.

Eddie and I did not know that the disease we read about in the *MMWR*, which did not resemble a sexually transmitted disease at all, was, in fact, mostly spread by sexual relations. We also did not know that it would eventually kill millions of people worldwide, becoming a leading cause of death in many countries, including the United States. Eddie and I had no way of knowing that it would claim the lives of many people we loved, including his own.

C.B.S.

Test Your Knowledge About HIV and AIDS

1. Behaviors such as sharing needles and syringes for injection drug use or having unprotected sex can transmit the human immuno-deficiency virus (HIV), even if neither partner is infected with HIV.

    ❏ True   ❏ False

2. Saliva, sweat, and urine of an HIV-infected person can transmit HIV because those fluids may contain the virus.

    ❏ True   ❏ False

3. Most babies born to HIV-infected women who do not receive any prenatal care or treatment are born with HIV infection.

    ❏ True   ❏ False

4. If a baby born to an HIV-infected mother has a positive HIV antibody test result, it means that the baby is infected with HIV.

    ❏ True   ❏ False

5. Even with preventive treatment during pregnancy, about one-third of infants of mothers with HIV infection will become infected.

    ❏ True   ❏ False

6. HIV, the virus that causes AIDS, is much smaller than the bacterium that causes chlamydia, and is smaller than a sperm cell, so latex condoms are less effective in preventing HIV transmission than in preventing chlamydia or pregnancy.

    ❏ True   ❏ False

7. Worldwide, most cases of HIV infection are related to sex between men and injection drug use.

❏ True   ❏ False

8. HIV infection is incurable and untreatable. Not much can be done to change the course of AIDS, which eventually and rapidly leads to death.

❏ True   ❏ False

9. Cases of HIV infection have been caused by the deliberate inappropriate disposal of needles used by infected injection drug users.

❏ True   ❏ False

10. Tests to see whether a person has antibody to HIV require a blood sample.

❏ True   ❏ False

11. The reason for the decline in death due to HIV at the end of the 1990s was people's increased awareness of HIV and their safer sex behaviors.

❏ True   ❏ False

12. Human papillomavirus infection, which causes cervical cancer, is more common than and just as deadly as HIV.

❏ True   ❏ False

Test Your Knowledge About HIV and AIDS

All of these statements are false; clarification of each statement is provided below. These are just a few of the common misconceptions about HIV and AIDS. At one time, some of these misconceptions may have been true. Information about this disease is constantly changing and being updated as more research is done. This book provides up-to-date information about HIV, AIDS, its misconceptions, and the prevention of this disease.

CLARIFYING COMMON MISCONCEPTIONS ABOUT HIV AND AIDS

1. Since HIV is a virus, nothing that two uninfected people do can result in transmission of HIV.

2. Although tiny amounts of virus and its antibody are detectable in urine and other body fluids of people with HIV, contact with tears, urine, and sweat from a person who is infected does not transmit HIV.

3. The risk of mother-to-child HIV transmission without treatment is about 25% to 40%; it is a huge risk, but is still not a certainty.

4. HIV antibody tests in babies reflect the mother's antibody, not necessarily the baby's own infection.

5. With treatment during pregnancy, the risk of mother-to-child HIV transmission can be decreased to less than 2%.

6. Testing sexual partners of people with HIV shows that most partners who do not use condoms become infected with HIV. However, partners who use condoms consistently are at much lower risk after similar numbers of sex acts with their infected partners, indicating that the degree of protection afforded by condoms is probably over 85% to

90%. This is probably higher than the degree of protection that condoms provide against some other sexually transmitted infections.

7. Worldwide, most HIV transmission is due to sex between men and women.

8. Treatments for HIV, while they do not cure the infection, are very effective in delaying the onset of symptoms for many years. The medicines, although very effective in delaying the onset of AIDS and progression to severe disease, do not cure HIV.

9. No HIV infections have been caused by used needles deliberately placed in public places.

10. HIV antibody testing can be done with saliva or urine samples.

11. The spectacular decrease in the number of new AIDS cases and deaths in the 1990s was due almost entirely to people receiving treatment with antiretrovirals to delay the onset of AIDS.

12. Infection with the human papillomavirus types that cause cervical cancer is very common, but most women with this infection never develop cervical cancer. Cancer can be prevented if changes are detected with Pap tests before they get too advanced. If cancer occurs, it can often be treated, and the patient cured, if detected in time.

1
History of the Epidemic in the United States

Between October 1980 and May 1981, five young, previously healthy homosexual men were treated in Los Angeles for **Pneumocystis carinii pneumonia**. This type of pneumonia is never seen in healthy adults. It usually affects people with severely weakened immune systems, such as recipients of transplanted organs. Organ recipients have to be treated with immune suppressive therapy so their immune systems will not **reject** the organ.

In the five young men, the pneumonia was very severe; two of them died despite treatment. All five of the men had previous or current cytomegalovirus infection and candida mucosal infection (thrush). Although cytomegalovirus causes severe disease and birth defects in babies if infected before they are born, it never causes serious disease in normal children or adults. Thrush is a nuisance disease for babies, but it is extremely rare in healthy adults.

In June 1981, the Centers for Disease Control and Prevention (CDC) published an article in their weekly newsletter, **Morbidity and Mortality Weekly Report**, on the five men and their cases. Soon after the report was published, information about the new disease spread quickly in the medical community.

All of the five men used illegal, inhaled drugs, popularly called "poppers," the slang term for amyl nitrite and similar drugs. The drugs come in glass vials that are broken open to release a vapor. This vapor is inhaled and, within seconds, causes the user's arteries to dilate, rushing blood to the heart and brain. These drugs are very addictive and occasionally cause heart attacks. Because all of the men with

14

GAY IN THE U.S.A.

The word **homosexual** means that a person is sexually attracted to members of his or her own sex. That is, a man is attracted sexually to other men or a women is attracted to other women. Homosexuality and heterosexuality (attraction to members of the opposite sex) are *sexual orientations*. Most people are **heterosexual**. However, researchers estimate that up to 10% of people, both men and women, are homosexual.

For centuries, sexual activity between persons of the same sex was illegal in the United States. Many homosexuals kept their orientation hidden. During the 1970s, many sexual behaviors changed. Sex became less of a taboo subject. Many people in the United States, particularly homosexual men, had sex with many partners. Condom use was common among heterosexuals for pregnancy prevention but it was not common among male homosexuals. This fostered the spread of sexually transmitted diseases (STDs) such as syphilis and HIV.

Although syphilis was easily diagnosed and treated with antibiotics, no one even knew HIV existed until homosexual men (and later, some heterosexuals as well) began to die of rare and mysterious diseases. HIV spread quickly through the male homosexual community in the 1970s and 1980s. **"Gays"** (male homosexuals) currently make up more than half of the men with HIV in the United States.

Gays introduced the concept of **"safer" sex** as a way to lower their risk of spreading HIV. They demanded streamlined testing of HIV medicines and equal rights for all people with HIV, including heterosexuals and children. Many male homosexuals volunteered to be in HIV studies. This helped scientists understand HIV and made effective treatment possible. In 2003, the U.S. Supreme Court struck down all laws that illegalized homosexual acts among adults. This was a step toward acceptance for the homosexual community.

Pneumocystis carinii pneumonia used the drugs, it was thought that perhaps these drugs harmed their immune systems.

When news of these five cases of *Pneumocystis carinii* pneumonia first reached the CDC, scientists at the CDC were already worried about unusual *Pneumocystis carinii* pneumonia cases. The medicine needed to treat *Pneumocystis carinii* pneumonia was not yet licensed by the **Food and Drug Administration (FDA),** so it was available only by request from the CDC's drug service. The CDC staff member who administered the drug service noticed with alarm that doctors from New York had requested the medicine to treat *Pneumocystis carinii* pneumonia in male patients who had been healthy homosexuals. Their immune systems had become weakened for no obvious reason.

After the first cases of *Pneumocystis carinii* pneumonia were reported, many other doctors reported rare, life-threatening infections in homosexual men, including brain infections due to yeasts and amoebae. Cancers, such as a severe, rapidly fatal form called **Kaposi's sarcoma** were also reported.

Kaposi's sarcoma is normally a rare, slow-growing skin cancer found mostly among older men. In affected homosexual men, it spreads rapidly, affecting not only the skin, but also internal organs (Figure 1.1). In July 1981, the CDC formed a Task Force on Kaposi's Sarcoma and Opportunistic Infections. Studies were conducted to determine how the new disease was spreading. The studies showed that the disease was probably infectious and sexually transmitted, and that it could also be spread by **transfusion** of tainted **blood products**, substances made from whole blood donated to blood banks by doners. No type of illegal drug was the culprit.

Cases of the new syndrome were also identified among infants born to women who had the disease or were at risk for it. The disease appeared to be related to swelling of **lymph nodes** that lasted for months. This swelling seemed to come before the disease. Although most cases continued

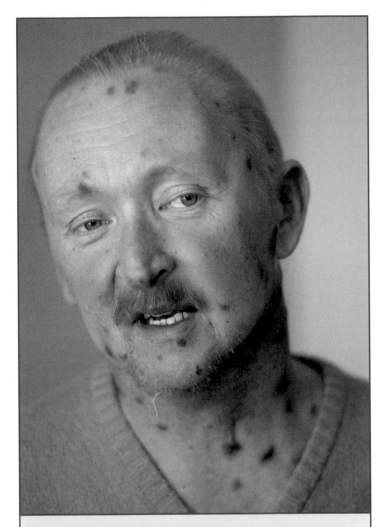

Figure 1.1 Shown here is a photo of Kaposi's sarcoma lesions on the face and neck of a man with AIDS. Kaposi's sarcoma is an opportunistic infection that can afflict individuals with weakened immune systems, such as those with HIV and AIDS.

to occur among men who had sex with other men, cases were also reported among other people, including women and children.

(continued on page 20)

HOW MEDICAL DETECTIVES CRACK A CASE

Investigating epidemics is not an epidemiologist's only job, but it is probably the most exciting. **Epidemiology** is the study of how a disease or unhealthy condition is distributed and spread in a population. Epidemiology works hand in hand with laboratory science, such as microbiology and virology. However, the techniques used in epidemiology are not laboratory techniques.

In epidemiologic terms, an **epidemic** is the occurrence of more than the expected number of cases of a disease, disease outcome, or other health event in a population. For some diseases, the expected number of cases is zero; a single case constitutes an epidemic. In 1981, the five cases of *Pneumocystis carinii* pneumonia (PCP) in young, previously healthy men were considered an epidemic because the expected number of cases of this disease in normal men is zero.

The techniques of epidemic investigation involve looking at characteristics of epidemic cases, to determine what people in the epidemic have in common. The epidemic investigators studied the behaviors and activities of these five men who contracted *Pneumocystis carinii* pneumonia, hoping to find out what was causing this epidemic. For example, one hypothesis was that the use of inhaled drugs might have damaged the patients' immune systems. Each hypothesis is then tested by comparing people who became ill ("cases") to those who did not (referred to as "controls").

A key first task for epidemiologists is to develop a case definition. "Cases" are the people with the epidemic disease. In the case of the men with PCP, the CDC's case definition of the new disease was, simply, "a person with *Pneumocystis carinii* pneumonia or severe Kaposi's sarcoma who did not have any reason to be severely immune suppressed." The CDC case definition was adopted quickly worldwide.

Physicians reported patients who matched the case definition to the CDC. Researchers also searched past records to determine if doctors had seen cases of the syndrome before they knew its significance. These efforts proved that the condition or disease was new; previous cases were virtually nonexistent.

The number of reported cases increased rapidly. CDC investigators led by Dr. Harold Jaffe carefully reviewed the details of the cases to see what they had in common. Then, with help from Dr. Jim Curran, then the director of the STD Division of the CDC, and many other scientists, they conducted a case-control study. This type of study compares people who have a disease (cases) to similar people who do not develop the disease (controls). Most of the patients who met the case definition and agreed to participate in the study were homosexual males.

The studies compared 50 cases to 120 matched controls. A long questionnaire was administered to each case and control by the epidemic investigators. The cases, many of them severely ill, tried to answer accurately the many, often very personal, questions about their lives. The controls answered the same questions. The investigators painstakingly recorded the answers.

As the results were evaluated, the investigators found that there were some significant differences between the case and control individuals. In the language of statistics, "significant" means that mathematically, the probability that a difference that extreme could be due to chance alone was very small. For example, the average number of male sexual partners per year for the cases was 61, more than twice that of controls (25). More than two-thirds of cases, but only about one-third of controls, had had syphilis in the past.

The case-control studies and other epidemiologic data showed that the new condition or "syndrome" was probably an infectious disease and spread sexually or through blood among injection drug users and blood transfusion recipients.

(continued from page 17)

In 1982, the Task Force adopted the term **Acquired Immunodeficiency Syndrome (AIDS)** for the new disease, dropping the term "gay-related immunodeficiency," which was used in the first months of the investigation. The following year, the Public Health Service used epidemiologic information about the disease to make recommendations on how to prevent AIDS. The Public Health Service advised that people should not have sex with or come in contact with the blood of people who were known or suspected to have AIDS. They asked people at risk for AIDS to avoid donating blood. They also helped **blood banks** develop safer blood products for people with **hemophilia**, a genetic (inherited) disease in which blood does not clot properly. Because hemophiliacs are at risk of bleeding to death, they frequently receive **blood transfusions** that provide them with the necessary clotting factor.

RISK FACTORS AND RISK GROUPS

Epidemiologic studies could not determine exactly what caused AIDS, but they did provide some information about the disease. They showed that people who had AIDS shared some characteristics. For example, male homosexuals who had AIDS were more than twice as likely to have had **syphilis**, a sexually transmitted infectious disease, in the past than other male homosexuals who did not have AIDS. These common characteristics are called **risk factors**; such characteristics are linked to a greater risk of having the disease.

As the disease was first being studied, researchers grouped people who seemed most likely to get AIDS into **risk groups**. These risk groups included men who had sex with men (mostly homosexuals), hemophiliacs, and injection drug users.

The Public Health Service recommendations in 1983 prompted many people to change their behavior. Men who had sex with men decreased their number of sexual partners and began using condoms more frequently. These changes helped reduce the risk of spreading AIDS. As the natural history of the infection with the human immunodeficiency virus (HIV), the virus that causes AIDS, became understood, it became clear that it takes years for full-blown AIDS to develop after HIV infection. Thus, the results of actions to decrease the risk of AIDS did not become visible in AIDS trends for years. But they became visible immediately in trends of other **sexually transmitted diseases** (STDs), diseases caused by organisms that are spread from person to person by or during sex.

During the 1970s, men who had sex with men were frequently infected with syphilis and other STDs due to unprotected sex with many partners. Starting in 1983, STDs in these men began to decrease dramatically. In 1985, Dr. Ward Cates, director of the CDC's Division of STD Prevention, remarked that the number of cases of syphilis might continue to decrease. He reasoned that "safe sex" (later known as "safer sex") introduced to prevent the spread of AIDS would decrease syphilis in the 1980s. He was mistaken about that prediction, as is discussed later. However, he warned in an August 1985 *Newsweek* magazine article about AIDS that "Anyone who has the least ability to look into the future can already see the potential for this disease being much worse than anything mankind has seen before."[2] He was right.

THE CAUSE OF AIDS IS DISCOVERED

In 1983, the cause of AIDS was discovered: **human immuno-deficiency virus**, or HIV. The discovery of HIV made it possible for scientists to develop a test for the virus, which helped to screen blood donors. This decreased the risk of HIV infection from a blood transfusion. Testing sites were established so people could get tested for HIV. The test showed that many individuals who had risk factors for AIDS but did not have AIDS, were already infected with HIV. Most people with positive tests had one or more risk factors. Researchers could conclude with some confidence that HIV was being spread through known **routes of transmission** (sexual intercourse or blood contact).

This was extremely reassuring, particularly to people who provided health care and other services to people with HIV. It showed that HIV was not easy to transmit. There was little risk to people caring for those with HIV, as long as precautions were taken to prevent blood or genital fluids from the patient coming into contact with the caregiver's blood or **mucous membranes**, membranes or linings of the body containing mucus-secreting glands.

In addition, much about the progress of HIV infection became clearer. HIV tests were positive in people who had no symptoms, had just lymph-node enlargement, had AIDS, and died of the disease. This suggested that HIV infection progressed through stages. It became clear that AIDS was actually a combination of HIV-caused **immunosuppression** and one or more **opportunistic infections**. Depending on where people with HIV lived and to what microorganisms they were exposed, AIDS could be cloaked behind tuberculosis, bacterial or amoebic food- and water-borne illnesses, fungal infections in the lungs or sinuses, or viral disease of the skin. As immune suppression became more severe, the number of opportunistic infections to which people with HIV could succumb grew. In the most severe stages, even organisms that never cause disease in normal people could cause death.

Scientists studied ways of treating HIV-related health problems in the various stages. They tried to prevent opportunistic infection, and tested drugs against the virus.

RISK OF HIV INCREASES

In the 1980s, several social changes increased the number of people who were at risk for infectious diseases, particularly syphilis, which promotes the spread of HIV. Before 1980, the federal government funded many programs, including programs to treat STDs and drug dependence, at low or no cost to patients. But in the 1980s, taxes needed for government support of public health programs were slashed. Clinic hours for people to get STD testing and treatment or **prenatal care**, the care of pregnant women, were cut in many areas. By 1985, many clinics closed altogether. The **infrastructure of public health**, which tends to be a safety net for those with little money and no private health insurance, was neglected. Poverty increased dramatically as unemployment rose. In some areas, the main source of income became drugs and prostitution, which promoted the spread of STDs, particulary syphilis. Syphilis was a risk factor for AIDS. If either the HIV-infected or uninfected sex partner had syphilis, the chance of HIV transmission was much greater. Increased numbers of untreated syphilis cases promoted the spread of HIV.

Syphilis can be treated with one injection of penicillin. By the early 1990s, the number of syphilis cases was greater than at any time since shortly after penicillin was discovered (Figure 1.2). Some doctors thought that HIV affected syphilis, making it harder to treat. But HIV was not what was causing the epidemic. The epidemic of syphilis was actually caused by social and economic factors that promoted drug selling and prostitution, and made early treatment of syphilis difficult for poor people. Cases of syphilis in men who had sex with men decreased, but the number of women with syphilis soared. During the nationwide syphilis epidemic, many infected pregnant women who had not received any prenatal care gave birth to babies with syphilis or who were born dead.

Of course, many people acquired not only syphilis, but also HIV. HIV rapidly followed the trends observed with the syphilis epidemic—widespread drug use and poverty, preferentially affecting mostly low-income heterosexuals. During the 1990s, **sexual transmission** of the virus among heterosexuals replaced **injection drug use** as the second leading route for spreading HIV (men having sex with other men remained the primary route of transmission).

Tuberculosis and HIV: Deadly Duo

Tuberculosis and HIV have much more impact together than the sum of their individual effects. This is called a **synergistic**

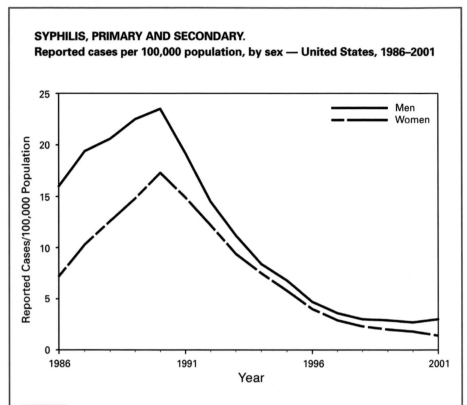

SYPHILIS, PRIMARY AND SECONDARY.
Reported cases per 100,000 population, by sex — United States, 1986–2001

The reported rate of primary and secondary syphilis increased slightly in the United States from 2.1 cases/100,000 population in 2000 to 2.2/100,000 in 2001. Among women, rates continued to decline, from 1.7 cases/100,000 women in 2000 to 1.4 cases/100,000 women in 2001, the lowest rate for women since reporting began in 1941. Among men, rates increased from 2.6 cases/100,000 men in 2000 to 3.0/100,000 men in 2001, the first increase since 1990.

Figure 1.2 During the late 1980s, the number of cases of syphilis per 100,000 persons rose dramatically, reaching levels not seen for decades. In the 1990s, syphilis declined rapidly, but started to increase again in males in 2001.

effect. However, even before HIV, tuberculosis was much more of a problem among the poor than the wealthy. Many factors tend to promote the spread of tuberculosis in poor people, and its progression to active, infectious disease.

Mycobacterium tuberculosis, the bacterium that causes tuberculosis, is spread in the air. Indoors, particularly where air circulation is poor, *M. tuberculosis* bacteria can stay suspended in the air for hours. Typically, poor people live in overcrowded environments. Also, many low-income people who live in the United States are immigrants from other countries where there are many people with infectious, untreated tuberculosis. If they were infected with tuberculosis before they immigrated, their infection may be **reactivated** after they arrive.

People living in poverty, particularly those who are homeless, are less likely to go to doctors when they are ill than other people are. Increases in unemployment and poverty during the 1980s resulted in a large increase in homelessness. Homeless shelters became overcrowded. Stricter laws required long prison sentences for drug use and resulted in prison overcrowding. Many people who were living in homeless shelters or who were incarcerated were infected with HIV. If infected with *M. tuberculosis*, they quickly developed active tuberculosis. In these overcrowded facilities, the spread of *M. tuberculosis* was rapid and efficient.

Months after being infected with *M. tuberculosis*, many prisoners and homeless shelter guests who progressed to active, infectious tuberculosis became the source of more infections. As a result, the United States experienced an upswing in the incidence of tuberculosis. This was startling after a long period in which the incidence of this disease had decreased dramatically. Epidemics of tuberculosis in HIV patients swept through prisons, homeless shelters, and city hospitals and hospices from 1988 to 1993.

Many people panicked, particularly those who were uninformed about the HIV epidemic. Some believed that AIDS was a punishment for "sins" such as homosexuality or drug use. Others suspected a sinister government plot to kill all gays, drug users, or black people, because these groups were, and still are, overrepresented among those living with HIV. Many people thought that HIV was spread through casual contact, and that any contact with people with HIV was dangerous. Some confused tuberculosis transmission with HIV

(continued on page 28)

HOW A BOY WITH HEMOPHILIA CHANGED OUR PERCEPTION OF HIV AND AIDS

Many of the people diagnosed with AIDS in the early days of the disease were members of groups of which many people disapproved. Because homosexual men and injection drug users were overrepresented among AIDS cases, some people thought that everyone with the disease belonged to those groups and should be shunned. Some of the hostility toward people with AIDS, however, was due to lack of knowledge regarding how it was transmitted. Fear that it was more contagious than anyone was admitting caused panic. Many people seemed to turn a blind eye to people living with HIV, until Ryan White came along (Figure 1.3).

Among the risk groups of people who were most likely to get AIDS in the early days of the epidemic were people with hemophilia. Hemophilia is an inherited disease where the body cannot make the proteins that cause blood to clot. Due to internal bleeding, hemophiliacs can die from bumps that do not even cause bruises in normal people. They also develop crippling diseases due to bleeding in their knees or other body parts. In the past, most hemophiliacs died during infancy or childhood. However, scientists discovered how to pool clotting factors from donated blood, and with transfusions of these clotting factors, hemophiliacs can live relatively normal lives.

Ryan White, a hemophiliac born in 1971, had been treated with clotting factors since shortly after birth. He received blood products from thousands of donors before AIDS was recognized and HIV testing of donors began. Like many hemophiliacs, he developed AIDS in the 1980s. When he was diagnosed with AIDS, he did not give up on his life or succumb to self-pity. Told he had only six months to live, Ryan decided to live as normal a life as possible and to continue going to school. However, many parents, teachers, and students at his Indiana school reacted with panic. Despite assurances that AIDS could not be spread through casual contact, Ryan was forced to use separate restrooms and drinking fountains, and disposable lunch trays and plastic utensils.

Even with these restrictions, many parents still wanted Ryan removed from the school. He became the target of teasing, vandalism, and death threats; a bullet was even fired into his home. The media publicized stories about "the AIDS boy," which inspired a flood of letters supporting Ryan. A movie about him prompted even more interest in the rights of people with AIDS. Elton John, a famous musician, befriended Ryan. Ryan and his mother used Ryan's fame to lobby for improvements in the lives of people living with HIV/AIDS.

Ryan did not live to graduate from high school. However, his story changed the way Americans viewed people living with HIV/AIDS. Shortly before he died in 1990, Congress passed the Ryan White CARE (Comprehensive AIDS Resources Emergency) Act to meet the needs of people living with HIV/AIDS. Congress amended and passed the Act again in 1996 and 2000. Various Ryan White CARE funds support health care and other services for people with HIV. Because of Ryan White's heroism and determination to live and learn despite his suffering, the nation's eyes were opened to the humanity of people living with HIV.

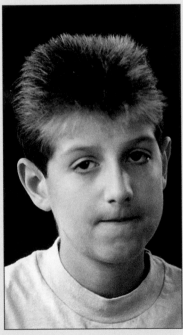

Figure 1.3 Ryan White (pictured here), a hemophiliac with AIDS, became a teenage activist, facing death threats and attempts on his life just to go to school. The government program for HIV treatment is named in his honor.

(continued from page 25)

transmission. Parent groups demanded that children with HIV be taken out of schools. In Florida, Indiana, and other states, the homes of children with hemophilia who were known or suspected to have HIV were burned to the ground in an attempt to intimidate their parents into moving and taking the children out of the schools.

HIV Becomes the Leading Cause of Death

For more than 40 years, injuries, heart disease, and cancer were the leading causes of death among people in the United States aged 25 to 44. But by 1994, for the first time in decades, an infectious disease, HIV, became the leading cause of death. Thousands of infants born to mothers with HIV infection were infected themselves in the early 1990s. Many of the uninfected babies became orphans as their mothers died from AIDS-related illnesses. In populations with a high prevalence of HIV, literally 50% or more died during the 1990s.

BREAKTHROUGHS IN THE PREVENTION AND TREATMENT OF AIDS

In the 1990s, ingenious biomedical and behavioral research and a renewed commitment to public health, supported by passionate AIDS activists, yielded breakthroughs in the prevention and treatment of HIV infection and AIDS.

The first antivirus HIV medication, **zidovudine** (azido-thymidine, AZT), was licensed. In 1993, scientists conducted a study comparing AZT to a **placebo**, or inactive pill, in pregnant women with HIV infection, to see if it would prevent HIV in the babies. Only 8% of the babies whose mothers had received AZT during pregnancy became infected. Of the babies whose mothers received a placebo, 26% were infected. AZT decreased the risk of a mother infecting her baby by more than two-thirds! The results of the study prompted the CDC to recommend that all pregnant women with HIV infection be offered AZT.

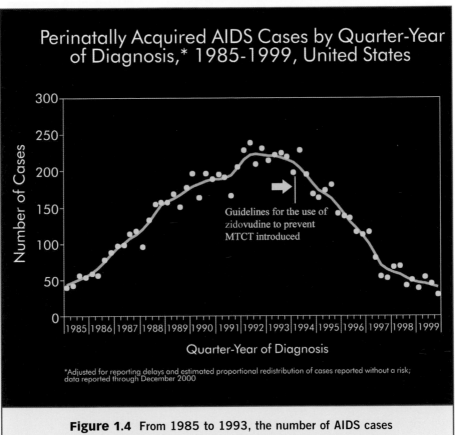

Figure 1.4 From 1985 to 1993, the number of AIDS cases among children attributed to the spread of HIV from mother to child soared to more than 1,000 per year. After pregnant women started getting tested for HIV and were offered treatment if they were infected, the number decreased by more than 90%.

Transmission of HIV from mothers to babies decreased by more than 90% (Figure 1.4).

Public health control programs responded to the increase in syphilis cases. They received funding, which allowed them to keep clinics open until everyone who had symptoms could be examined and treated. People who did not have symptoms, but who had had sex with someone with syphilis, were screened, sometimes in their own communities, and offered treatment.

People in communities with high syphilis rates were offered free blood screenings. By 2000, the number of syphilis cases had decreased by more than 90%, to the lowest level in United States history (refer again to Figure 1.2).

Thousands of people with HIV, including many homosexual men, volunteered for randomized **placebo-controlled studies** to test **antiretrovirals**. Antiretrovirals interfere with certain activities that HIV needs to reproduce. In the past, the process to get medicines approved for general use was very long. Activists urged the Food and Drug Administration (FDA) to streamline the process for getting new drugs approved for use. Although the process is now much quicker, it still takes years to thoroughly test any product used to prevent and treat HIV. During testing, some drugs that had looked promising were found to be unsafe or ineffective, so they were discarded or modified. Other drugs provided important breakthroughs in how we prevent and treat HIV infection.

The self-sacrifice of the volunteers paid off. By the mid-1990s, the number of antiretrovirals approved by the FDA jumped from one (AZT) to more than 10. In 1996, at the International HIV Conference, combinations of these drugs were described as **highly active antiretroviral therapy (HAART)**. Use of AZT alone did not help AIDS patients. But the drug combinations appeared to impact HIV infection greatly. While the combinations worked best if used earlier in the course of **immunodeficiency**, their use even helped patients with advanced AIDS. In fact, some people who were near death recovered after taking HAART, returned to work, and are living healthy, normal lives today.

As these drugs became more widely used, the number of HIV deaths decreased. By 1996, HIV dropped to fifth place as a cause of death in young adults in the United States (Figure 1.5). However, it should be noted that, to date, there is no cure for HIV infection. All of the persons successfully treated with combinations of antiretrovirals are still

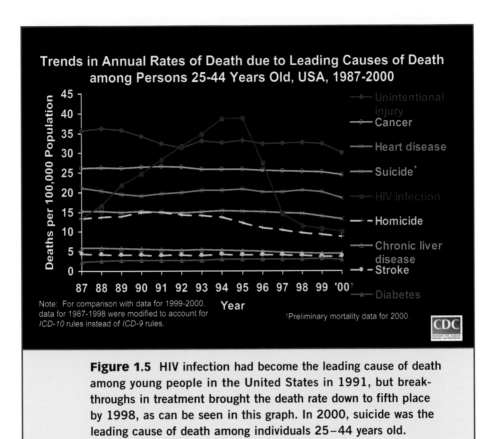

Trends in Annual Rates of Death due to Leading Causes of Death among Persons 25-44 Years Old, USA, 1987-2000

Note: For comparison with data for 1999-2000, data for 1987-1998 were modified to account for *ICD-10* rules instead of *ICD-9* rules.

†Preliminary mortality data for 2000.

CDC

Figure 1.5 HIV infection had become the leading cause of death among young people in the United States in 1991, but break-throughs in treatment brought the death rate down to fifth place by 1998, as can be seen in this graph. In 2000, suicide was the leading cause of death among individuals 25–44 years old.

infected with HIV, can infect others, and can eventually die from HIV infection.

Many men who had sex with men increased their efforts to promote safer sex. Following their lead, heterosexuals also reduced their number of sexual partners and increased condom use. Adolescents delayed the start of sexual activity, and those who were sexually active used condoms. As a result of these efforts, HIV transmission decreased during the 1990s. The estimated number of new HIV infections decreased from about 80,000 to 40,000 per year.

Lawyers worked with people in jails and prisons who had HIV, tuberculosis, or both. They argued that the rights of people who were infected with *M. tuberculosis* after they were incarcerated had been violated. The lawyers believed that contracting a possibly fatal disease in prison was cruel and unusual punishment, which the United States Constitution forbids. They argued that it was the responsibility of prison administrators to ensure that the health of the inmates was protected. The Supreme Court agreed, and now all prisons and jails must provide treatment for ill inmates, and protect those who are not ill from becoming infected.

Other advocates successfully lobbied to have AIDS classified as a **disability**, and worked to have laws passed to protect disabled people from discrimination in housing and other services. People who were disabled because of AIDS became eligible for services and support, like those offered to people disabled by other illnesses or injuries. These developments made getting an HIV or AIDS diagnosis far less of a disaster. People with HIV became less likely to become jobless or lose their rights.

TROUBLING TRENDS IN THE 21ST CENTURY

In the 21st century, a new trend emerged. Gone is the panic of the 1980s. Researchers have developed effective treatments to slow down the progress of HIV infection. The downside of this is that some people in various risk groups do not think HIV is a serious problem anymore. Some have reverted to unsafe sexual practices that increase the risk of transmitting HIV and other infections. Others are too young to remember how deadly HIV can be.

In 2001, the number of reported syphilis cases increased for the first time in 10 years. In 2001 and 2002, outbreaks of syphilis among men who have sex with men occurred, often involving men who knew they had HIV. Clearly, HIV transmission is probably increasing again in these populations. The rate of death due to HIV is not decreasing anymore. For the first time in years, the number of AIDS cases increased in 2001.

Since 1995, most cases of AIDS have been among African Americans. Because African Americans and Latinos with HIV are more likely than whites to be uninsured and poor, they have not benefited as much from the breakthroughs in HIV treatment. They are less likely to be diagnosed with HIV early in the course of their HIV infection, when the medicines work best. They are more likely to die from HIV-related illnesses than others with HIV.

2

The HIV Pandemic: A World of Difference

HIV ORIGINS AND IMPACTS IN AFRICA

Because HIV infection has reached epidemic proportions in many regions of the world, it is referred to as a **pandemic**. However, no countries have suffered as much from the ravages of HIV/AIDS as African countries south of the Sahara Desert.

Scientists believe that HIV emerged in Africa in the late 1950s. This was probably due to contact with **simian immunodeficiency virus** (SIV) types that can cause disease in humans. These viruses could be found in the blood of nonhuman primates, such as apes and monkeys, that were hunted for food. These primates are slaughtered with knives and axes, and then prepared for cooking. During this process, humans often come in contact with the animal's blood. The first infections of humans with immunodeficiency viruses probably occurred when primates were used for food.

Hundreds of thousands of blood specimens obtained during surveys and studies around the world have been tested for HIV **antibody**. The earliest blood specimen that was positive for HIV antibody was obtained in 1959 from a man in central Africa. HIV tests of blood specimens collected in the 1960s and 1970s show that HIV spread very little until the late 1970s in Uganda and the Republic of the Congo. Botswana and South Africa had relatively low rates of HIV infection in the early 1990s, affecting less than 5% of the population. However, social and economic factors led to poverty, high-risk sexual behaviors, collapse of public health infrastructures, and spread of sexually transmitted diseases that promote the spread of HIV. HIV infections increased dramatically. By 1999, almost one-third of adults in those countries were infected with HIV.

Immunodeficiency viruses have always been quite difficult to transmit. Injection drug use was virtually unheard of in Africa during the 1950s and 1960s. Transfusions were rarely used, except for treatment of severe malaria. Mosquito control programs and antimalaria medicines were reducing the threat of malaria. Most Africans lived their entire lives in rural areas where sexual mores were conservative. They did not move around very much. Thus, HIV infection was sporadic in Africa for decades, as in North America. There was not enough transmission to sustain an epidemic, or to even recognize HIV's emergence.

However, in the late 1970s and 1980s, in central Africa as in North America, many changes occurred that resulted in rapid spread of this epidemic (Figure 2.1). In sub-Saharan Africa, where the highest levels of HIV infection are seen now, very little transmission occurred until the 1980s. Epidemic transmission was fueled by thousands of cases of sexually transmitted diseases, which promoted HIV transmission and social upheavals that decreased public health services. HIV epidemic transmission first followed strife in Uganda and the Central African Republic (now Democratic Republic of the Congo). Famine, dictatorship, and warfare forced many rural people from their homes to work in large cities, on the road as truckers, and into prostitution. Separated from family and with little expectation of survival, many people abandoned the traditional customs that had protected them, not knowing that they might become infected with HIV.

REGIONAL HIV/AIDS STATISTICS AND FEATURES, END OF 2002

Region	Epidemic started	Adults and children living with HIV/AIDS	Adults and children newly infected with HIV	Adult prevalence rate (*)	% of HIV-positive adults who are women	Main mode(s) of transmission (#) for adults living with HIV/AIDS
Sub-Saharan Africa	late '70s early '80s	29.4 million	3.5 million	8.8%	58%	Hetero
North Africa & Middle East	late '80s	550 000	83 000	0.3%	55%	Hetero, IDU
South & South-East Asia	late '80s	6.0 million	700 000	0.6%	36%	Hetero, IDU
East Asia & Pacific	late '80s	1.2 million	270 000	0.1%	24%	IDU, hetero, MSM
Latin America	late '70s early '80s	1.5 million	150 000	0.6%	30%	MSM, IDU, hetero
Caribbean	late '70s early '80s	440 000	60 000	2.4%	50%	Hetero, MSM
Eastern Europe & Central Asia	early '90s	1.2 million	250 000	0.6%	27%	IDU
Western Europe	late '70s early '80s	570 000	30 000	0.3%	25%	MSM, IDU
North America	late '70s early '80s	980 000	45 000	0.6%	20%	MSM, IDU, hetero
Australia & New Zealand	late '70s early '80s	15 000	500	0.1%	7%	MSM
TOTAL		42 million	5 million	1.2%	50%	

* The proportion of adults (15 to 49 years of age) living with HIV/AIDS in 2002, using 2002 population numbers.
# Hetero (heterosexual transmission), IDU (transmission through injecting drug use), MSM (sexual transmission among men who have sex with men).

Figure 2.1 Epidemic spread of HIV started in North and South America, Europe, the Caribbean, and sub-Saharan Africa in the late 1970s and early 1980s. In the late 1980s, North America and Asia began experiencing epidemics. In the early 1990s, a huge epidemic broke out in the former USSR, Eastern Europe, and central Asia.

HIV was recognized as an epidemic much later in Africa than in North America. Tuberculosis was more frequent in Africa, so the immune systems of many African people with HIV and *M. tuberculosis* infection never had a chance to become suppressed enough to develop *Pneumocystis carinii* pneumonia or the other more unusual opportunistic infections associated with HIV. Instead, they developed tuberculosis, a common problem in Africa, and died of it without ever being suspected of having the new disease. However, once HIV **antibody tests** became available, it was easier for public health workers to determine how much HIV was spreading in Africa.

PATTERNS OF EPIDEMIC SPREAD

Although the effect of HIV has been felt worldwide, especially in developing countries, the epidemic has been most severe in southern Africa, Asia, and the Caribbean, particularly Haiti. There are two patterns of epidemic transmission. The epidemic of HIV/AIDS in developed countries has been driven greatly by HIV spread in men who have sex with men, injection drug users, and, to a lesser degree, by heterosexuals. As a result, most cases occur among men. This pattern of epidemic spread is termed Type I.

In most of the developing world, particularly Africa, injection drug use and sex between men has played a relatively small role in spreading HIV. Most cases have been transmitted when infected men have sex with women, or when infected women have sex with men. This pattern is called Type II. In these countries, the number of cases among women is about as high as among men. Because HIV infection is more easily spread from men to women than from women to men, the number of infected women may be slightly higher than that of men in some of these countries.

In some countries, such as South Africa, and even some areas of the United States, there is a high degree of segregation by racial or ethnic group or socioeconomic status. In those countries, Type I and Type II HIV occur in tandem, with Type I in more industrialized populations and Type II in less industrialized populations of the country.

HIV/AIDS in poor countries and in poor communities in developed countries is part of a vicious cycle. Poverty and lack of preventive medical services and treatment for infectious diseases increase transmission of HIV. HIV then robs countries of their most productive population—young adults—who are the most likely to become infected by

HIV/AIDS PATTERNS OF TRANSMISSION WORLDWIDE

In 2002, about 42 million people worldwide were living with HIV/AIDS; 38.6 million were adults, and about 50% of these were women. Another 3.2 million were children under 15 years of age. Five million new infections of HIV occurred in 2002, along with over 3 million deaths due to HIV/AIDS (Figure 2.2).

Most of the human population lives in nonindustrialized developing countries, where HIV is spread primarily by sex between men and women. In many of these countries, HIV infection is generalized, meaning that it is not confined to people who have specific risk factors as defined in the early investigations.

The continent where the highest proportion of the population is infected with HIV is Africa. More than 75% of AIDS deaths occur in Africa, and in some countries, more than one out of every four persons is sexual transmission. Illness and death among these young adults leads to more poverty and fewer services and treatments, which, in turn, further increases the transmission of HIV. Aided by high rates of sexually transmitted diseases and other infections that increase a person's chance of becoming infected with HIV, HIV transmission is extremely efficient in poor populations. HIV infection is responsible for undoing progress that had been made to increase life expectancy and decrease child mortality in Africa and other areas in the developing world. It is believed that children born today in many African countries have far less chance of reaching their first birthday than they did in the 1980s.

believed to have HIV infection. However, HIV/AIDS is spreading very quickly in large Asian countries, such as China and India, so there may be more Asians than Africans living with HIV/AIDS in the next decade. Injection drug use plays an important role in spreading HIV in some Asian countries.

The region that has the second highest proportion of inhabitants infected with HIV is the Caribbean. More than 3% of adults in Haiti, the Dominican Republic, and Panama are believed to be infected.

In most developed countries, including Canada, United States, Western Europe, and Australia, most men with HIV infection have had sex with other men. In these countries, HIV spread is far less generalized, and the proportion of the general population that is infected tends to be lower.

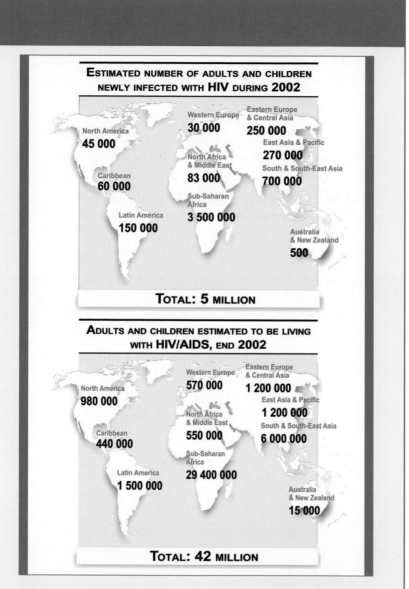

Figure 2.2 In 2000, more than 5 million adults and children became infected with HIV (top). Of the 42 million people living with HIV infection in 2002, almost 30 million live in Africa (bottom).

RESPONDING TO THE CRISIS

Some leaders have been slow to respond to the crisis. Unconvinced that prevention of HIV infection is important, they have limited people's access to condoms or antiretrovirals that reduce mother-to-child transmission, further worsening the situation.

The situation for people living with HIV/AIDS in developing countries is far worse than for those in wealthier countries. In many areas, education is extremely limited. Most people do not know about microorganisms, and their understanding of disease is minimal. They may believe that HIV/AIDS is a punishment for bad things that a person or his/her parents have done. Some people who know they have not done anything "wrong" to deserve this disease may think that it is due to magic or that someone who hated them made them sick.

In many developed countries, including the United States, the availability of antiretroviral drugs (see Chapter 6) has dramatically changed the impact of HIV infection. However, in most developing countries, antiretrovirals are not available, so mortality rates have not decreased. Among international aid organizations, there has been controversy about whether complex medical treatments such as antiretrovirals can be introduced in health-care systems so poor that they cannot even deliver routine, simple interventions such as immunizations.

This has led to an emphasis only on prevention of HIV infection in many developing countries. But the possibility that antiretroviral treatments can be provided in areas where they are most urgently needed in the developing world is finally being explored. Dr. Paul Farmer, M.D., Ph.D., who has worked for many years at Harvard University and in a clinic he helped found in Haiti, invented a concept that he calls "complex health interventions in poor settings"

(CHIPS). Applying CHIPS, he has proven that treatment for HIV with highly active combinations of three or more antiretrovirals can be used in Haiti, the poorest country of the Western Hemisphere, lengthening patients' productive, symptom-free lives.

In the late 1990s, Brazil became the first developing country to guarantee free antiretroviral treatments to all people living with HIV infection. Using antiretrovirals made locally or provided through trade agreements with drug companies, Brazil can offer various combinations of antiretrovirals at low cost to the government. As a result, death from HIV infection has decreased dramatically in Brazil.

Dr. Farmer's successes, and the success of Brazil's program in the production and distribution of antiretrovirals, have proven that the poor need not wait decades for the benefits of technological breakthroughs. The U.S. government has directed all government agencies to ensure that all HIV prevention and care efforts in developing countries include treatment with antiretrovirals.

Africa remains the hardest-hit continent. But the alarming spread of HIV is also occurring elsewhere, particularly in Asia and the former Soviet Union. Originally, HIV/AIDS mostly affected Thailand, where an epidemic raged during the early 1990s. However, a very successful campaign to promote condom use and other prevention strategies greatly reduced HIV transmission in Thailand. In India, sexual transmission of HIV is increasing. Although they have much smaller numbers of affected people, the developing regions of the Caribbean have, after Africa, the highest proportion of their population living with HIV. In some countries, such as Brazil and Haiti, researchers, advocates, and people living with HIV/AIDS have come together to respond to the crisis. In other countries, however, poverty, ignorance, and other crises continue to divert attention from priority health issues, particularly HIV.

3

The Virus

THE ANATOMY OF A VIRUS

In order to understand how HIV spreads through a population and how this epidemic can be thwarted, we must first understand the virus itself. HIV, like all viruses, is composed of a core and a protein coat (Figure 3.1). Its **genetic material** is stored in its core. The genetic material of all animals, including humans and bacteria, is coded in the **nucleus** of the cell. The chemicals in the nucleus that maintain this genetic code are called **nucleic acids**. Other **microorganisms** (living beings that cannot be seen with the naked eye) and all other animals and plants have two types of nucleic acids: **ribonucleic acid** (**RNA**) and **deoxyribonucleic acid** (**DNA**). Viruses, however, have either DNA *or* RNA, but not both. HIV's nucleic acid is RNA, so HIV is called an RNA virus. The protein coat (**capsid**) carries the chemicals that make it possible for HIV to enter cells.

Once inside a cell, HIV uses the cell's machinery to produce energy and reproduce itself. Using an **enzyme** called **reverse transcriptase**, HIV makes a DNA copy of its RNA and inserts it into the host cell's DNA. This is the reverse of the normal order. Normally, inside the cells, DNA codes for RNA, a process called **transcription**. Viruses that can make a DNA copy from RNA are called **retroviruses**, because they reverse the usual process.

HIV's RNA carries codes for only nine **genes**, sections of nucleic acids that determine a trait or characteristic of a living being. (In comparison, a human being has about 30,000 genes, which determine the color and texture of hair, gender, and everything else that is inherited.) HIV's nine genes code for viral proteins that have specific functions. Three of these genes, *gag, pol,* and *env,* contain information needed to make structural proteins for new virus particles. The *env* gene, for example, codes for a big

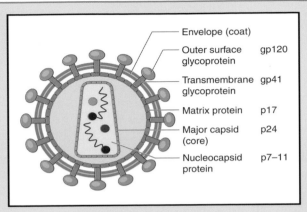

Envelope (coat)

Outer surface   gp120
glycoprotein

Transmembrane   gp41
glycoprotein

Matrix protein   p17

Major capsid   p24
(core)

Nucleocapsid   p7–11
protein

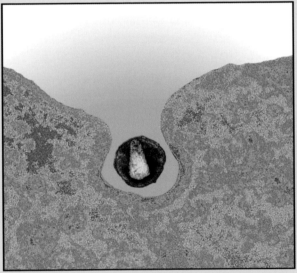

Figure 3.1 The culprit exposed: HIV virus. At the core of
the HIV virus is the capsid that contains strands of DNA.
When the virus infects a healthy cell, this DNA is copied into
the now unhealthy cell's existing DNA and new virons form and
leave the cell (for more on the HIV life cycle, see page 58.)
The DNA-carrying nucleocapsid is protected by the envelope
(the innermost layer and several layers of protein membranes).
On the surface of the envelope are glycoproteins, which
attach to the surface of a cell during infection and cause the
cell to draw the virus inside (bottom).

DISCOVERY OF THE VIRUS
THAT CAUSES AIDS

When Dr. Robert Gallo, honored as the codiscoverer of the human immunodeficiency virus, first came to the National Cancer Institute at the National Institutes of Health (NIH) in 1965, he had no idea that he would be staying for over 20 years. He planned to return to a medical school eventually, where he could teach and do clinical work as well as basic research. But he became addicted to research and studying viruses that cause cancer. He saw basic research translated into life-saving treatment at the NIH Clinical Center, the clinical research hospital of the NIH. He was thrilled to see children actually being cured of leukemia, a cancer of the blood, for the first time.

Dr. Gallo eventually decided to look for a human retrovirus. Many in the scientific community thought human retroviruses simply could not exist, even though other animals acquired retroviral infections. Dr. Gallo discovered the first known human retroviruses, human T cell leukemia viruses I and II, shortly before the first AIDS cases were recognized in 1981. In 1982, Gallo proposed that a retrovirus caused AIDS.

Dr. Luc Montagnier, a native of France who has been an active researcher in virology for over 35 years, discovered how RNA viruses multiply. Throughout the 1970s, he studied RNA viruses that caused cancers. In 1983, as head of the Viral Oncology Unit at the Pasteur Institute in Paris, he discovered a retrovirus in damaged lymph node samples from a patient with AIDS. Because the retrovirus was in all the damaged lymphatic tissues, he suspected that this was the retrovirus behind AIDS. He called it Lymphadenopathy (swollen lymph nodes) Associated Virus. Gallo called it Human T cell Leukemia

Virus III. In the 1980s, virologists agreed to call it human immunodeficiency virus (HIV). Researchers found HIV in many tissues from people with AIDS by growing it in culture. Many other researchers using their techniques also cultured the virus, and photographed it using electron microscopy.

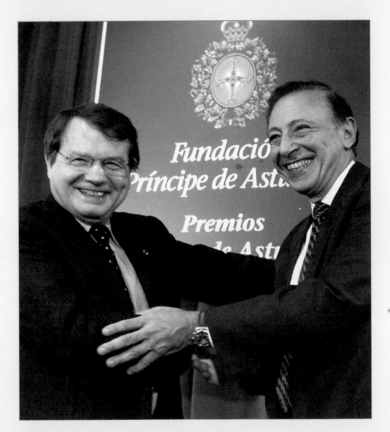

Figure 3.2 Doctors Robert Gallo (right) and Luc Montagnier shared the Nobel Prize for their discovery of the virus that causes AIDS, which came to be known as human immunodeficiency virus (HIV). Here, they are honored for their research.

(continued from page 44)

precursor protein called **glycoprotein** 160 (gp160), which is broken down by a viral enzyme to form gp120 and gp41, the components of the viral envelope. The numbers 160, 120, and 41 are the molecular weights of these proteins. Three regulatory genes, *tat, rev,* and *nef,* and three auxiliary (helper) genes, *vif, vpr,* and *vpu,* contain information needed to make proteins that HIV uses to infect a cell and make new copies of itself. The protein for which the gene *nef* codes, for example, appears to be necessary for HIV to replicate efficiently. The protein that is encoded by *vpu* helps release new virus particles from infected cells.

Retroviral infections do not kill the cells that they infect. However, many of them cause tumors (cancers). The family of retroviruses to which HIV belongs does not cause cancers directly.

HIV's subfamily is called **Lentivirinae** (or "slow" virus) because these types of retroviruses cause chronic infections that progress slowly. Lentiviruses are very specific as to what type of host they can infect. HIV only infects humans and chimpanzees—not dogs, cats, or other animals. Two HIV types infect humans, HIV-1 and HIV-2. HIV-2 causes a much milder disease than HIV-1. Throughout this book, the term HIV will refer only to HIV-1. Table 3.1 lists examples of immunodeficiency viruses (IVs), the species they affect, and the disease caused by each.

HIV Needs Special Conditions to Survive

Compared to many other viruses, HIV is fragile. Unlike some viruses, such as hepatitis B, which can be dried and survive for at least a week, HIV cannot tolerate drying. It also dies if exposed to prolonged heat. Antiseptics and disinfectants like chlorine and alcohol quickly kill HIV outside the body. Even people who have very high quantities of HIV in their blood cannot spread HIV by using public toilets or baths because the virus cannot stay alive for long outside of the

Table 3.1: The Retroviruses, Subfamily Lentiviruses

HOST	VIRUS	DISEASE CAUSED
NON-PRIMATES		
Cat	Feline IV	Feline AIDS (mild disease)
Horse	Equine infectious anemia V	Anemia
NONHUMAN PRIMATES		
African Green Monkey	Simian IV (SIV)agm	Simian ("monkey") AIDS
Rhesus macaque	SIVmac	Simian ("monkey") AIDS
Sootey mangabey	SIVsm	Simian ("monkey") AIDS
Chimpanzee	SIVcpz	Simian ("monkey") AIDS
HUMANS		
Males and females	HIV-1, identical to SIVcpz	AIDS
Males and females	HIV-2, identical to SIVsm	Less severe AIDS

body. However, once the organism has entered the body, it is much harder to kill.

THE IMMUNE SYSTEM

To understand how HIV causes acquired immunodeficiency syndrome (AIDS), it is necessary to understand the human immune system. Human beings are in constant contact with millions of microorganisms, many of which could cause serious or fatal disease. Every human being, however, has a defense system to protect it from invasion. This defense system includes the immune system, a complex defense run by white blood cells that protect us from infection and disease. The body's defenses also include barriers, such as skin and mucous membranes that block microorganisms from entering the body.

When humans come in contact with viruses, bacteria, or other microorganisms, these organisms may take up residence in some part of the body, such as the mucous membranes of the mouth or nose, without interfering with organ functions.

LIVING IN A BACTERIAL (AND VIRAL, AND FUNGAL . . .) WORLD

Human beings live surrounded by and covered inside and out with a vast array of microorganisms (Figure 3.3). About 5% of the body weight of an average human consists of microorganisms. A person who weighs 120 pounds is hauling about 6 pounds of bacteria, fungi, and other microscopic beings.

Most of these microorganisms are harmless to us as long as they stay on the skin or linings (mucous membranes) of the respiratory, gastrointestinal, or genital organs, where they are kept in tight control. If they stray deeper into the body, they trigger the immune system into producing cells that fight and kill the foreign organisms.

Most encounters with bacteria, viruses, or other microorganisms do not result in infection. Even if they do, many infections do not actually cause infectious diseases. Infectious "disease" means that an infection has actually disrupted the normal functions of a body organ or organs. These are often prevented because humans have several lines of defense that limit damage of invading microorganisms.

This is called **colonization**, which is usually harmless to the host. Sometimes, however, microorganisms do not stop at colonization. They multiply to great numbers using the resources of the human host. They may produce toxic products as a way of invading the host or as a by-product of their growth, and may damage or kill cells.

This process of **infection** does not always lead to organ malfunction, but it can. When infection proceeds to the point that one or more organs actually malfunction, the process is

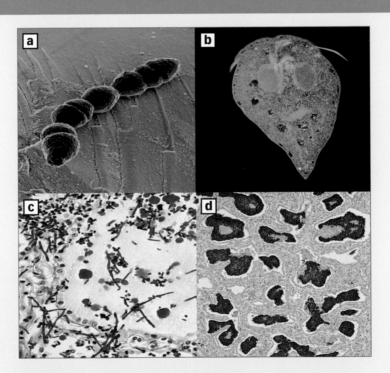

Figure 3.3 Bacteria such as *Streptococcus pneumonia* (a), amoebae such as *Giardia lamblia* (b), and fungi such as *Candidia albicans* (c) and *Pneumocystis carinii* (d), can cause severe disease or death in vulnerable hosts.

called an **infectious disease**. Infectious diseases may be **acute**, with symptoms appearing rapidly after infection, or **chronic**, resulting from infections that progress over months to years.

The immune system contains many kinds of white blood cells, including:

- **Granulocytes**—When there is no acute infection, about one-third of the white blood cells are granulocytes, cells with small grains that release chemicals that kill some microorganisms.

- **Lymphocytes**—The general defense system includes lymphocytes (cells in a clear fluid called **lymph**) that circulate in the body. Some lymphocytes are called **natural killer (NK) cells** because they do not have to be primed or prepared in any way to destroy invaders.

- **Macrophages**—Other white blood cells that are non-specific defenders are called *macrophages* (meaning "big eaters"). These either stay in areas where there are frequent invasions of microorganisms (such as the mouth) or are summoned by white blood cells to clean up debris after a skirmish.

The body's immune system is a sophisticated and very specific monitoring system that recognizes foreign materials (**antigens**). When cells of the immune system encounter an antigen, they spring into action by a process called **activation**. The type of antigen determines how the immune system responds.

Most of the cells of the immune system are lymphocytes. Lymphocytes work in one of the two arms of defense of the immune system. These two arms are antibody-mediated (humoral) immunity and cell-mediated immunity.

Antibody-Mediated Immunity

Antibody-mediated immunity is provided by antibodies in the body's fluids, such as blood and lymph. It involves lymphocytes that originate in the bone marrow and travel into the blood and lymph vessels. Because these lymphocytes go directly from the bone marrow to the blood without maturing in another organ, they are called **B lymphocytes** or **B cells** (the *B* stands for "bone"). B cells respond to antigens by becoming potent antibody-producing cells. Antibodies neutralize **toxins.** They are very effective against attacks by many types of bacteria.

Cell-Mediated Immunity

The other arm of the immune system is **cell-mediated immunity**, which depends on lymphocytes that go from the bone marrow to the **thymus**. The thymus is an organ found in the chest below the thyroid gland. There, lymphocytes are programmed to respond to activation. Because they have to pass through the thymus to become functional, they are called **T lymphocytes** or **T cells** (the *T* stands for "thymus"). When activated, T cells are the main defenses against cancers, viruses, and most parasites and fungi. They respond to antigens by producing **cytokines**. Some antibodies cannot be made without cytokines. T cells also respond by producing **chemokines**, which attract cells that will destroy invading microorganisms.

T cells have chemicals on their surfaces called **cluster designation (CD) markers.** These markers distinguish lymphocytes from one another. Humans have almost 200 CD markers. When T cells leave the bone marrow to travel to the thymus, they have two types of CD markers: CD4 and CD8. In the thymus, they lose one and keep the other. Which one they keep determines what types of activities they can perform. Most lose CD8, so they have only CD4 on their surface. Because they have CD4 only, they are called CD4-positive (CD4+) T cells. Macrophages also have CD4.

CD4+ T cells

CD4+ T cells are the most important cells for cell-mediated immunity, and are called **helper T cells**. In people with healthy immune systems, most white blood cells are lymphocytes, most lymphocytes are T cells, and most T cells are helper T cells.

When helper T cells are activated, they produce cytokines that create **inflammation**, an organized, effective attack against invaders. Inflammation draws various types of cells to the site where the antigen has invaded. Helper T cells also recognize organ **transplants** from another person as foreign, and stimulate an inflammatory response to reject the transplanted organ. If a person needs an organ transplant, such as a kidney, liver, heart, or lung, he or she is given drugs that

WHITE BLOOD CELLS

Before a baby is born, the liver produces stem cells, which are the precursors (ancestors) of all the cells in the blood. These include precursors of red blood cells and two of the major types of white blood cells: granulocytes (cells with small grains) and lymphocytes (lymph cells) (Figure 3.4).

Granulocytes that patrol the blood looking for micro-organisms are often called **polymorphonuclear** ("many shaped nucleus") **leukocytes** (PMLs), because their nuclei are bent into different shapes. They are differentiated by the colors that the granules retain when exposed to dye. If the granulocytes pick up eosin, a red stain, they are called *eosinophils* ("loves red").

The granules in polymorphonuclear leukocytes contain chemicals that are particularly effective for different broad types of microorganisms. *Neutrophils* ("loves neutral color," which, in the terms of cell staining, is pinkish) kill bacteria, while eosinophils kill parasitic worms. Other cells that come from the granulocyte precursors are *macrophages* ("big eater") and *dendritic* ("has tentacles") cells. These two types do not patrol the body but mostly remain in tissues often exposed to microorganisms so they can grab many types of microorganisms if they try to invade.

slow down the work of the helper T cells. These medicines are called suppressants of cell-mediated immunity (immuno-suppressants). People who take these medications to suppress cell-mediated immunity have very few helper T cells. As a result, they become very vulnerable to many serious infections.

Helper T cells also recognize parasites, viruses, and fungi as foreign. They produce cytokines to create intense attacks to destroy them. Some antibodies produced by B cells are only effective if helper T cells produce cytokines in response to an antigen.

Lymphocytes are a type of leukocyte found in the blood and lymph nodes. Some lymphocyte stem cells develop in the bone marrow into what are called "natural killer," or NK, cells. NK cells zero in on all foreign things and kill them.

However, other lymphocyte stem cells develop in the bone marrow to become mature B cells, which can turn into plasma cells. Plasma cells make antibodies. Other lymphocytes mature in the thymus. These are called T cells, and they make cytokines and other chemicals. B and T lymphocytes can mount attacks to very specific invaders. Unlike granulo-cytes, which attack broad types of microorganisms (bacteria or parasitic worms), B and T cells can tailor their response to very specific species of microorganisms. They can make antibodies to a specific virus, such as chicken pox or the chemical that a bacterium makes that causes tetanus (lockjaw). Lymphocytes patrol the blood and the lymphatic system, which consists of lymph nodes and other lymphoid tissues that are strategically placed to be able to drain areas of the body where there is most exposure to microorganisms. Lymph nodes in the neck, sinus, and tonsils protect the mouth and nose. Nodes in the groin stop organisms from coming through injuries in the feet, anus, or genitals.

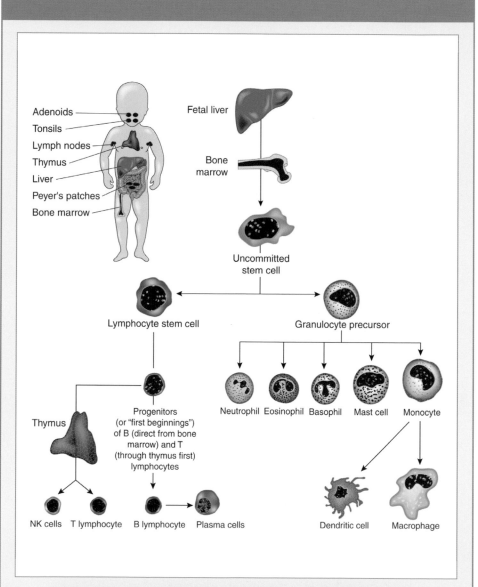

Figure 3.4 The liver in the fetus makes stem cells, from which all the cells of the immune system descend. In babies and young children, immune tissues such as adenoids and the thymus are very prominent. This figure illustrates the different immune cells that arise from stem cells.

CD8+ T Cells

T cells that lose their CD4 in the thymus and keep only their CD8 are called CD8+ T cells. Cells that have CD8 on their surfaces make cytokines that slow down inflammation once invaders have been controlled. Otherwise, the inflammatory response may actually continue and damage normal tissues. Because they slow down the **immune response**, CD8+ T cells are called **suppressor T cells**. Normally, helper T cells outnumber suppressor T cells, so the ratio of helper to suppressor cells should be more than one to one. When activated, other T cells are programmed to become **cytotoxic (cell-killer) T cells,** which destroy damaged, infected, and cancerous cells.

Primary Response of the Immune System

The first time an antigen is encountered, the response it causes is called a **primary response**. If it provokes a response from the antibody-mediated arm of the immune system, the primary response will include antibodies specific to the invader; in just a few days, "first-draft" antibodies will be noticeable in the host's blood. In several weeks, streamlined, final, specific antibodies will be generated. If the antigen activates the cell-mediated immune system, it will provoke the release of cytokines.

Secondary Response of the Immune System

When the same antigen is encountered again, a powerful **secondary response** overwhelms the invader, because the cells "remember" this foreign invader, recognize it, and quickly eliminate it. Usually, the human host is not even aware that the antigen has been encountered again because the secondary response is so efficient. Lymphocytes that have been primed to recall an antigen are called **memory cells**. This response is called **anamnestic**, meaning "did not forget." Lymphocytes that have never seen an antigen are called **naïve cells**.

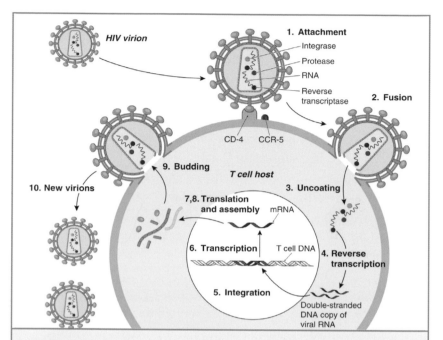

Figure 3.5 Shown here is a schematic of the HIV life cycle.

1. HIV binds to the T cell by attaching to "handles." These include CD-4 and chemokine co-receptor (CCR)-5.

2. The membrane of the virus (envelope) and the cell membrane fuse.

3. HIV injects its capsid, with its nine genes coded by its RNA, as well as its enzymes, and it is uncoated in the cytoplasm of the cell.

4. Reverse transcriptase, an enzyme in HIV, copies the viral RNA into viral DNA.

5. Viral DNA enters the nucleus, and viral integrase enzyme splices the viral DNA into the T cell's DNA.

6. The cell's nucleus uses the viral DNA inside of its own DNA as a template for making RNA for a new virus, and for making big, inactive proteins for new viruses.

7, 8. The new viruses are trimmed into individual active proteins by protease enzymes.

9. The new virus particle buds out of the cell, assembled, just taking with it a tiny bit of cell membrane for itself. It does not damage the cell, which stays busy making more HIV.

10. The new virus goes on to infect another cell.

THE HIV LIFE CYCLE

HIV must successfully pass through several steps in order to infect a person (Figure 3.5). These steps, as described more fully in the rest of the chapter, are:

- Binding to the cell;

- Fusing with the cell membrane;

- Replicating itself with reverse transcription;

- Releasing new viruses from the cell.

HIV Must First Bind With a Cell

To be able to infect a cell, HIV has to bind to the cell. The binding works only if the virus can attach to a cell at a specific binding site, or "handle." HIV can only attack cells with the appropriate type of binding site. The CD4 surface molecules of helper T cells are the main binding sites for HIV. All primate lentiviruses use CD4 as a binding site to bind to T cells or macrophages. HIV and other lentiviruses seek out T lympho-cytes, so they are called T *lymphotropic* (meaning they "go toward lymph cells").

However, CD4 is not the only binding site that HIV uses. A second receptor is also needed. HIV uses **chemokine co-receptors** (**CCRs**) present on the surface of some cells. CCRs normally assist helper T cells, providing a place for cytokines and other chemicals to attach, and then directing them to microorganisms to which they should bind. HIV's membrane gp120 binds first to CD4, and then to CCR-5 or another CCR. HIV can also use CCRs in cells in the **cervix** (mouth of the womb) and the large intestine as binding sites.

HIV Cannot Bind With Some Cells

Genetics determines which CCRs are on cells that have CD4 on their surfaces. Most people inherit normal "wild-type" genes that code for CCR-5 on cells with CD4; HIV can easily infect

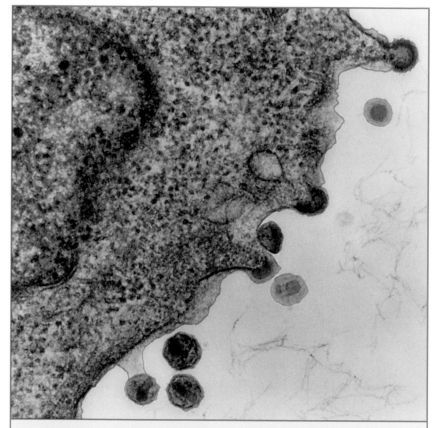

Figure 3.6 The virus at work: This electron micrograph shoes the HIV virions budding and leaving an infected cell.

their cells. However, about 1% of people of Northern European ancestry do not have any CCR-5. They inherited **mutations** from both parents for the gene that codes for CCR-5, so they cannot make it. If exposed to HIV, they seem to be much less likely to get HIV infection than other people.

People who inherit one gene mutation for CCR-5 and one "wild-type" (normal) gene make some CCR-5. They can become infected, but do not progress to immunodeficiency as quickly after HIV infection as those with two CCR-5 "wild-type" genes.

After binding, **fusion** takes place and the membranes of HIV and the cell combine. Then, the virus makes copies of itself. During reverse transcription, the enzyme called reverse transcriptase makes a DNA copy of HIV's RNA; this DNA is inserted into the host cell's DNA as a **provirus**, which remains quiet in the cell's genetic material until the cell is activated. The immune system does not recognize it as foreign. If the cell is activated, the genes in the provirus will code for HIV proteins while the host cell's genes code for human proteins.

The HIV proteins, created in large, inactive form, are broken down into active proteins by enzymes called **proteases** and are organized into an incomplete, immature **virion**, or virus particle. The virion buds from the cell, taking with it a tiny piece of cell membrane, and forms a mature virus particle, which can infect another cell (Figure 3.6).

If the cell does not become activated and does not divide, no virions are made. This state of lying low inside the cell's DNA coincides with the 5 to 10 years that HIV infection is clinically **latent** (inactive). The patient has no symptoms but can transmit HIV to others during this time. However, if and when the cell is activated, the provirus will spring back to life inside the cell's DNA.

4

From Infection to Death: How HIV Causes AIDS

Not only do microorganisms tend to be selective about the hosts they infect, but most are selective about how they are spread. The first step in infection, introduction of HIV into a human host, is exposure to HIV. Every new HIV infection, like every new infection of any type, begins with the microorganism. HIV needs a route of transmission, or a way to get into an uninfected person. People who are not infected with HIV cannot spread HIV.

ROUTES OF TRANSMISSION

HIV is spread through several routes of transmission. HIV cannot survive drying or high temperatures. Thus, transmission requires transfer from the infected host to another host's tissue, where there will be cells with the binding sites that HIV needs to infect a cell, without drying or heating in between.

As described in this chapter, the most common routes of exposure to HIV are:

- Direct contact with an infected person's blood;

- Sexual contact with an infected partner;

- From mother to child.

Direct Contact With Infected Blood

The most efficient way to spread HIV is by injecting it into the blood of an uninfected person. A transfusion from an infected donor with viral particles in his or her blood is very likely to transmit the infection to an uninfected recipient. A tiny amount of blood in a needle or syringe used by an infected injection drug user may contain many viral particles. If an uninfected person uses this needle or syringe to inject something into his or her vein or skin, these viral particles can easily enter the bloodstream.

Experiments with *Rhesus* monkeys, which develop a disease very much like human AIDS, have been done using a combination of the human immunodeficiency virus (HIV) and simian immunodeficiency virus (SIV) called SHIV. These experiments have shown that few viral particles are needed to transmit the SHIV to uninfected monkeys if injected into the blood. However, if a monkey has the virus placed in its rectum, it takes a higher quantity of the viral particles to establish infection. If the virus is placed in the vagina, even more virus is needed to establish infection.

Sexual Contact With an Infected Partner

Sexual transmission is the way that HIV is most commonly spread worldwide. Unbroken skin is virtually impenetrable by HIV. Sex acts that involve only contact between normal, unbroken skin surfaces (e.g., hand to genital) do not transmit HIV. The tissues of the genitals, mouth, and eyes are much less resistant than the skin of the arms and hands. However, even these tissues, called mucous membranes, are formidable barriers to HIV. When they are intact, the cells are arranged so that they constitute a strong defense. The likelihood that HIV will be transmitted through sex depends on several factors (see "Will Sexual Exposure to HIV Lead to Infection?" on page 65).

Mothers Passing the Infection to Their Babies

Mothers can spread HIV to their babies during pregnancy, while giving birth, or by breastfeeding. Babies are generally very well protected from most organisms in the mother's blood, including HIV, by a normal, healthy placenta, particularly in the first months of pregnancy. Thus, most transmission occurs during the last months of pregnancy or delivery.

Most transmission from mother to infant occurs when the baby is exposed to the mother's blood during birth. During delivery through the vagina, the baby is covered with the mother's blood, and will have blood in the eyes, mouth, and other mucous membranes. The mother's blood also enters nicks and scratches that the baby may sustain during the birth process, particularly if the baby is premature, with skin that is not yet completely developed.

The likelihood of the mother transmitting HIV to her baby depends on several factors, including:

- How much virus is in her blood;

- How much contact there is between the baby's skin and mucous membranes and the mother's blood;

- How much inflammation there is in the placenta, allowing cells with HIV to come in contact with the baby;

- Whether the baby is premature.

In general, the risk of a mother with HIV transmitting infection to her child is estimated to be somewhere between 20% and 40%. After birth, if the mother breastfeeds, her milk may carry HIV to the baby. Because the mucous membranes of the baby are still quite delicate for months after birth, the risk of HIV transmission is greatest if the mother has a high amount of HIV in her milk, if she has infection or inflammation in her breasts or nipples, with inflammatory cells that carry HIV, or if the baby has inflammation or infections in its mouth or gastrointestinal tract.

Most women with HIV who deliver babies in the United States take antiretroviral medicines. In many of those women, no virus can be found in the blood. Their babies have less than a 2% chance of being infected. If the baby is delivered by

caesarean section, so that the baby is not exposed to the mother's blood or genital fluids, the risk can also be very low. If the baby is born uninfected and is fed with formula instead of breast milk, the mother's infection will not be transmitted to the baby.

WILL SEXUAL EXPOSURE TO HIV LEAD TO INFECTION?

A person's chance of becoming infected with HIV increases with the number of times he or she is exposed to the virus. The higher the number of exposures, the more likely it is that infection will occur. However, even one exposure can result in infection. Many variables influence how vulnerable a person is to developing an HIV infection after one exposure, including:

- Which partner in a sexual encounter is infected;

- The levels of HIV in the infected partner's blood or genital fluids;

- Whether either partner has other infections that could be making cells with "handles" that HIV needs more of;

- Whether either partner has infections or open sores or cuts that reduce the effectiveness of mucous membrane barriers;

- Whether a person is more resistant to infection.

Which Partner in a Sexual Encounter Is Infected

Certain factors affect whether an uninfected person will become infected with HIV through having sex with an infected partner. If the infected partner is the one who inserts his penis into the uninfected partner's vagina, mouth, or rectum, it is more likely that HIV will spread to the uninfected partner than if it is the *uninfected* partner who inserts his penis into the infected partner's vagina or rectum. If *either* partner has a cut, nick, sore, or irritation on his or her genitals, even if these are not visible to the naked eye, the chance of spreading the infection increases greatly.

Levels of HIV in the Infected Partner's Blood

In addition, the higher the concentration of virus in the infected partner's blood or genital fluids, the more likely that the exposure will lead to HIV spread. Although there is antibody in many body fluids, antibody is made by the host's B cells in response to HIV and cannot spread the disease. Only the virus itself can establish infection. The amount of virus found in saliva, urine, or **mucus** without blood is not enough to be able to spread infection.

The concentration of HIV in an infected person's blood changes during the course of the infection. During some stages of the disease, the HIV level is very high. At other times, it is very low. During those periods when it is low, however, HIV still resides in the body's cells, slowly reproducing. When people have very high levels of virus in their blood, the virus is also often found at high levels in other body fluids, such as genital fluids, but minimal, if any, virus is found in the sweat, urine, or tears. Sexual partners of people with high levels of HIV in their bloodstreams are very often infected, unless they have consistently taken measures to reduce their risk.

Other Infections Can Make the Immune System More Vulnerable

Other infections may also increase the chance of transmitting or being infected with HIV because the person's immune system is already being challenged. In the partner with HIV infection, other infections cause helper T cells to become activated to fight those infections. While reproducing, they make billions of new HIV particles, as do their daughter T cells. In the uninfected partner, other infections increase the number of helper T cells, and the numbers of "handles" per T cell, making these cells that are the main target of HIV readily available (the infections **upregulate** HIV, as discussed later on page 70). Of course, infections that cause ulcers or sores on the genitals or rectum, or that bring vulnerable white blood cells to the area where genital fluids with HIV will be found, dramatically increase the risk of spread.

Some People Can Resist HIV Infection

Some individuals appear to be resistant to HIV infection even after having unprotected sex with an infected partner many times. Some of these **highly exposed, persistently seronegative (HEPS)** (uninfected) individuals do not have the genes that code for CCR-5 or other binding sites that HIV needs to infect cells. Despite many exposures to HIV, they will not become infected.

Other research suggests that HEPS individuals may be more likely to be infected with **"hepatitis" G virus** than people who do get infected when they are exposed to HIV. The "hepatitis" G virus does not cause hepatitis or any other disease, but it may provide protection against infection by other microorganisms.

People who repeatedly have protected sex with those who have HIV infection, such as the wives of men infected with HIV who consistently and correctly use latex condoms, are also very unlikely to become infected.

FIRST SYMPTOMS OF HIV INFECTION

Nobody can tell immediately whether he or she has been infected with HIV after an exposure. About one in three people who are infected with HIV experience some symptoms, such as a rash, fever, or swollen lymph nodes, a few weeks after becoming infected. During those days, the person's blood will contain virus particles and the number of CD4+ T-cells dips. These symptoms are called **retroviral** or **seroconversion syndrome**. This name is given because at the time when symptoms are present, the antibody against HIV can start to be detected in the patient's **serum**, so his or her serum will be converted from negative to positive.

As the antibody becomes detectable, the number of CD4+ T cells increases again and the amount of virus in the blood decreases. For years, the antibody appears to control the HIV, and the number of CD4+ T cells remains high enough to fight off opportunistic infections.

THE "VIRAL LOAD"

After the development of the test to detect antibody to HIV, there was a lot of interest in trying to see if detection of actual virus material could be improved. Viral cultures and tests for antigens were negative in many people with HIV infection who were clearly infecting others. There was a need for tests that actually detected HIV better and more easily than the available tests.

In 1983, Dr. Kary Mullis, a DNA chemist in California, invented a process he called polymerase chain reaction, or PCR. PCR could make copies of a strand of DNA, an invention for which he later received the Nobel Prize. PCR uses the same molecules that nature uses for copying DNA: two "primers," one to mark each end of a DNA segment to be copied. An enzyme called polymerase walks along the segment of DNA, "reading" its code, and makes copies (or "polymerizes") the DNA strand using DNA building blocks (nucleic acids). As Dr. Mullis later wrote in *Scientific American*, "Beginning with a single molecule of the genetic material DNA . . . PCR can generate 100 billion similar molecules in an afternoon. The reaction is easy. . . . The DNA . . . can be pure, or it can be a minute part of an extremely complex mixture of biological materials, (it) may come from . . . a tissue specimen . . . from a drop of dried blood at the scene of a crime, from . . . a mummified brain. . . ."[3]

A few years after this invention, in 1987, Dr. Clyde Hart, a young virologist and expert in viral genetics at the CDC, used a version of PCR to detect HIV RNA in the blood of persons with HIV infection. He detected HIV RNA in persons with no

THE PROGRESSION OF HIV INFECTION

The length of time between getting the infection and developing symptoms of the disease depends on a number of factors. For most adults in the United States and other industrialized countries, the time between HIV infection and death is more

symptoms, those with mild symptoms, and those who had advanced AIDS. PCR also detected HIV proviral DNA (the DNA that an infected cell makes based on HIV RNA and integrates into its own DNA) in 94% of persons in the study. Dr. Hart and his colleagues predicted that because of the rapid and sensitive nature of PCR in detecting HIV, the PCR technique might be good for monitoring antiviral treatment.

In 2003, Dr. Hart stated that at the time he published his findings in 1988, he had no idea just how widely used PCR was going to be for HIV treatment and research. Neither did Dr. Mullis. Literally millions of PCR tests for the amount of HIV per milliliter of blood ("viral load" tests) are performed worldwide to monitor whether people with HIV infection need or are responding to treatment. HIV PCR tests have shown that immediately after infection, there is usually a large quantity of HIV nucleic acid in the blood of the infected person, and that as antibody is made against HIV, the viral load decreases, usually to the point that it is not detectable by the PCR test. Then, as HIV infection progresses, an increase in the blood viral load accompanies the decrease in the number of CD4+ (helper) T cells, severe immunodeficiency, and death.

HIV PCR tests have also shown that infected persons are most likely to spread infection when their blood viral load is very high. However, the viral load in semen and other genital fluids can be very high even if no HIV is detectable in the blood. Tests have also shown that when people with HIV infection take combinations of antiretrovirals, the viral load can decrease to an extent that it is no longer possible to detect it in the blood with PCR.

than 5 years, generally about 10 years. However, babies infected before or during birth usually have signs of serious immuno-deficiency within months of birth. The amount of virus that infects the person appears to be important. Some HIV strains may also be far more aggressive than others. Babies, especially premature babies, are exposed to a large quantity of virus relative to their size. Similarly, people who are infected via blood transfusions or are accidentally stuck with a syringe that has a lot of blood (a quarter teaspoon or more) probably get many millions of virions; the amount of time from their infection to the time of onset of disease may be small. In contrast, the amount of HIV that is transmitted to adults having consensual sex may be small, so it often takes longer to become ill.

Sometimes, having other infections can upregulate HIV. Dutch researchers have found that bacterial infections can encourage HIV **replication** through upregulation of chemokine receptors on T cells. Upregulation means that a bacterial infection will increase the number of co-receptors that HIV can use to fuse to the T cell. Upregulation also increases the number of infected T cells that are reactivated. Because only activated T cells produce virions, activating T cells that have provirus in their DNA increases the amount of virus in the blood.

HIV does not actually kill T cells as it leaves them. Often, T cells that are infected by HIV and are reactivated become HIV factories, meaning that they produce huge quantities of HIV particles, without appearing to be damaged. However, this does not fully explain why, at a certain point in the course of infection, the ability of the immune system to protect itself is over-whelmed. It is unclear why this happens. In order for HIV to survive, the immune system must not break down too soon after infection; if the system remains viable for several years (even more than a decade in some people), the HIV has more opportunity to replicate itself into billions of HIV virions. These virions can then spread the HIV infection to many more hosts.

WHAT HAPPENS WHEN HIV DISEASE GOES UNTREATED?

HIV establishes infection only if the virus connects with a cell that has receptors ("handles") that allow it to bind ("stick") to the cell. At this point, HIV can insert its RNA into the cell's cytoplasm. For several weeks, the cell will make virus RNA as it makes its own DNA and divides, making more HIV. HIV will spread throughout the lymphoid tissues of the body as the immune system tries to contain it. Within six to eight weeks, there will be enough HIV in the blood to be detectable in the tests described in the box on page 68. As more HIV finds and takes over more and more CD4+ T cells, the number of CD4+ T cells decreases. One of every three people who are infected with HIV will get fever, body aches, enlarged lymph nodes, or rash during this period. The rest will have no signs of the infection.

B cells then start making antibody to HIV. When HIV antibody appears in the blood, there is a drop in the amount of HIV in the blood. The number of CD4+ T cells increases again. After a period that generally lasts several years, the amount of HIV in the blood starts to climb again and the number of CD4+ T cells decreases. If people have latent *Mycobacterium tuberculosis* infection, it reactivates to active tuberculosis. Otherwise, patients may have no symptoms until the number of CD4+ T cells falls below about 300 cells per milliliter of blood. They may start feeling weak, tired, or feverish, or may get stubborn yeast infections, pneumonias due to bacteria, and recurrences of fever blisters. If a person goes untreated and is infected with *Pneumocystis carinii*, he or she will develop *Pneumocystis carinii* pneumonia as the number of CD4+ T cells continues to decrease.

The number of CD4+ T cells continues to fall until the infected person is susceptible to even more normally harmless organisms. If the person survives, he or she will gradually lose weight, have diminished brain function, and eventually die, usually about 10 years after first becoming infected with HIV.

At some point, the amount of HIV DNA in the host's blood increases, and the number of CD4+ T cells declines. The number of CD4+ T cells remains the most important indicator of immune response. Once that number declines, many organisms that normally could do no harm or only limited harm attack. This results in opportunistic infections.

OPPORTUNISTIC INFECTIONS

The cell-mediated immunity in the body protects against many infections, especially those caused by viruses, yeasts, and bacteria of the genus *Mycobacterium*, which includes *Mycobacterium tuberculosis* and other species. HIV-infected individuals' cell-mediated immunity becomes weakened. Therefore, they are vulnerable to becoming infected by many other microorganisms and developing serious or fatal diseases. All opportunistic infections that are seen in people whose immune systems are weakened by HIV can also be seen in people whose immune systems are severely weakened by other causes, including genetic diseases or medicines used to suppress the immune system, such as those to prevent rejection of transplants. Common opportunistic infections include esophagus (food tube) infections due to *Candida* yeast species; blindness, meningitis, and other severe diseases from cytomegalovirus or usually harmless amoebas; and *Pneumocystis carinii* pneumonia. Many of these illnesses are never seen in people with normal immune systems. Others, such as mucous membrane *Candida* infections (thrush), are seen in people with normal immune systems, but they are more likely to be severe or fatal in immunodeficient people.

Tuberculosis Is the Most Common Opportunistic Infection

Worldwide, tuberculosis is the most common opportunistic infection related to HIV. Tuberculosis is caused by the bacterium *Mycobacterium tuberculosis*. If a person with HIV has untreated *M. tuberculosis* infection, his or her first oppor-tunistic infection will generally be tuberculosis.

Almost a third of people on Earth have *M. tuberculosis* infection, but only about 10% of them actually develop active tuberculosis if they have a normally functioning immune system. Their T cells keep *M. tuberculosis* confined in lymph nodes, where they can do no harm. However, virtually all people with *M. tuberculosis* infection whose cell-mediated immunity is weakened will progress to active tuberculosis, many will have unusually severe disease, and all will die of tuberculosis if not treated.

Medicines have been available for years to prevent *M. tuberculosis* infection from progressing to tuberculosis and to treat active tuberculosis. Nevertheless, in many developing countries, including some in sub-Saharan Africa and in some populations in the United States, many HIV-related deaths are due to tuberculosis. When individuals with HIV develop active tuberculosis, they are no longer said to have just HIV infection; they are then classified as having AIDS. Of course, many people who progress to tuberculosis do not have HIV. Their immune system will just be weakened because they are babies, very old, or have other chronic diseases, such as diabetes, or stressors, such as malnutrition, homelessness, or other factors.

People with HIV infection generally do not develop other serious opportunistic infections, such as *Pneumocystis carinii* pneumonia, until the number of CD4+ T cells they have is very low. However, progression to tuberculosis is common even in untreated people with HIV who have high numbers of CD-4+ T cells.

Most people with HIV infection who develop tuberculosis are infected with *M. tuberculosis* in late childhood or adoles-cence before they are infected with HIV. After a mild illness (primary tuberculosis), which most do not even notice, they recover. The infection still exists in the body, but it is kept in check by cell-mediated immunity. In this state, the infection is called latent because it appears to become inactive. However, once HIV causes immunosuppression, the infection becomes reactivated, and infected people go on to develop active tuberculosis. In people with HIV infection, tuberculosis is far more likely to spread beyond the lungs, causing disease in many other organs, including the kidneys, bones, heart, and intestines.

Because HIV is very likely to cause reactivation, it is recommended that all people with unknown HIV infection status who develop tuberculosis be offered HIV testing. Almost one-third of people in the United States and more than half of people in some developing countries who develop active tuberculosis have HIV infection. Conversely, many people with HIV infection have latent *M. tuberculosis* infection that, if untreated, will develop into tuberculosis.

In the 1990s, epidemics of tuberculosis in people with advanced cell-mediated immunosuppression due to HIV showed how fast people progress from infection with *M. tuberculosis* to active tuberculosis. These people were infected by a person with unrecognized active tuberculosis while in specialized wards for people with HIV infection. In crowded prisons or homeless shelters, people with active tuberculosis spread infection to people with HIV. The patients whose immune systems were weakened by HIV developed symptoms of tuberculosis about four months after their exposure and presumed infection with *M. tuberculosis,* without any latency period. Their tuberculosis was caused by a **strain** that was very resistant to antituberculosis drugs, so treatment was ineffective. They died of HIV-related tuberculosis (AIDS) within five months.

Other Infections Resulting From Cell-Mediated Immune Deficiency

However, if HIV-infected adults do not have *M. tuberculosis* infection, they are not likely to develop severe opportunistic infections until their CD4+ T cell count decreases. As this number declines, the person becomes susceptible to infection by many more organisms. When the T cell count is very low, many microorganisms that are usually harmless can kill the patient.

There are no early warning signs of severe cell-mediated immunity deficiency. The signs and symptoms that signify AIDS are many and varied, reflecting the variety of micro-organisms to which patients are exposed; most people with AIDS develop only a few of the myriad opportunistic infections that fit the case-definition of AIDS.

Pneumocystis carinii *pneumonia*

The most frequent opportunistic infection in people with HIV infection in the United States is *Pneumocystis carinii* pneumonia. People with normal immune systems who are infected with *P. carinii*, the organism that causes this type of pneumonia, can easily fight the organism and do not become ill at all. Many, if not most, adults are infected with *P. carinii*. It is not sexually transmitted, and is commonly found in soil and other harmless substances. Most people who have infection with *P. carinii* do not even know they have it. However, people with HIV who are infected with *P. carinii* and are not treated to prevent the pneumonia when they become immunosuppressed quickly progress to cough, chest pain, low oxygen in the blood, and severe disease. Without treatment, they often die.

Kaposi's sarcoma

Certain cancers caused by viruses, such as Kaposi's sarcoma and cervical cancer (cancer of the cervix, the opening of the uterus), are also opportunistic infections that can arise after the number of T cells decreases. Kaposi's sarcoma is caused by one of the herpes viruses (human herpes virus 8), which can be spread sexually. This type of cancer develops when thousands of new, tiny blood vessels start growing unchecked, generally in the skin and mucous membranes of the mouth, nose, or eye. In people with normal immune systems, this process is slow and rarely life-threatening. In people with HIV/AIDS, the lungs, liver, stomach, intestines, and lymph nodes also may be involved, often causing severe disease or death.

WHAT, EXACTLY, IS AIDS?

Because much has been learned about how HIV infection progresses, the definition of "AIDS" has changed from the original definition used in 1981. In 1993, an expanded definition was developed that included all the knowledge available to classify HIV infection into three categories, or levels, of numbers of CD4+ T cells, and three categories of clinical (illness) severity (A,B,C).

CLINICAL CATEGORIES

CD4+ T Cells	A	B	C
Greater than 500	No or mild symptoms or signs of immunodeficiency	Moderately severe symptoms or signs of immunodeficiency	AIDS Conditions
200 to 499	No or mild symptoms or signs of immunodeficiency	Moderately severe symptoms or signs of immunodeficiency	AIDS Conditions
Less than 200	AIDS	AIDS	AIDS Conditions

AIDS is diagnosed in any person with HIV who has, or has ever had, a CD4+ T cell count of less than 200 cells per milliliter, or any one of the 26 "C" conditions, which include:

- Active tuberculosis

- Invasive cancer of the cervix (mouth of the womb)

- Repeated bouts of bacterial pneumonia

Cervical cancer

Cervical cancer is caused by certain types of **human papilloma-virus**; other types of this virus can also cause common skin warts or genital warts, which are sexually transmitted. About 14% of women in the United States are infected

- Repeated bouts of *Salmonella* infection

- *Pneumocystis carinii* pneumonia

- Kaposi's sarcoma

- Cancer of the lymph nodes in the central nervous system in people younger than 60 years

- Candidiasis (yeast) infection of the esophagus, trachea, bronchi, or lungs

- Infections anywhere other than the lungs with other fungi such as *Cryptococcus* or *Histoplasma*

- *Cryptosporidium* (an amoeba) infection lasting longer than a month

- *Cytomegalovirus* (CMV) infection of any organ except the liver, spleen, or lymph node

- Genital herpes or mouth fever blisters that last for more than one month or that are in the bronchi, lungs, or esophagus

- Brain lesions caused by *Toxoplasma gondii*, an amoeba, in patients over one month old

- Direct brain damage

- Wasting due to HIV

with the papillomavirus that causes most cases of cervical cancer. Even in women with normal immune systems, these infections may progress to cervical cancer (although they generally do not). But women with HIV infection who are also infected with these viruses are very likely to quickly develop cervical cancer.

Other cancers

Other cancers that threaten people with HIV are probably not caused by viruses; these cancers may be related to loss of the T cell functions related to monitoring and destroying cells whose growth appears to be abnormal.

Diseases at the End Stage of AIDS

During the most severe stage ("end stage") of AIDS, and probably throughout the course of infection, the virus directly damages some organs, particularly in infants. HIV damages the brain and can result in mental retardation in children and **AIDS dementia** in adults. Most people with severe AIDS get diarrhea, which is sometimes caused by opportunistic infections or HIV damage to the intestine. Many people with AIDS experience loss of appetite, nausea, and sometimes vomiting, along with diarrhea. Dehydration and weight loss often occur in AIDS patients. People who lose a significant amount of weight are said to have "wasting" or "slim" disease.

EPIDEMIOLOGIC SYNERGY: WHEN ONE DISEASE IS MADE WORSE BY ANOTHER DISEASE

The term *synergy* means that when two or more things are combined, their effect is greater than would be expected by just adding the effects of each. For example, when two drugs work synergistically, the results are stronger than just the effects of one drug plus the effects of the other drug. Similarly, some infectious diseases enhance each other's disease-causing effects (Figure 4.1). For example, the progress of HIV infection is

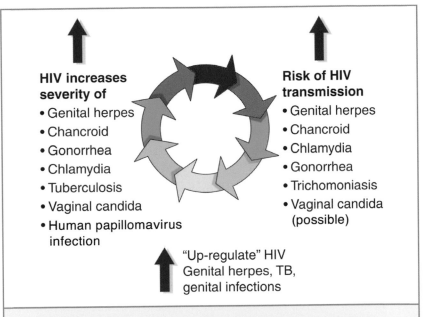

HIV increases severity of
- Genital herpes
- Chancroid
- Gonorrhea
- Chlamydia
- Tuberculosis
- Vaginal candida
- Human papillomavirus infection

Risk of HIV transmission
- Genital herpes
- Chancroid
- Chlamydia
- Gonorrhea
- Trichomoniasis
- Vaginal candida (possible)

"Up-regulate" HIV Genital herpes, TB, genital infections

Figure 4.1 In a type of "synergy," genital sexually transmitted diseases and other infections increase the risk of acquiring or transmitting HIV. HIV also makes these other infections far more severe.

greatly accelerated by infection with *M. tuberculosis* and herpes simplex virus. Herpes simplex 1 and 2 are DNA viruses of a large class that cause chronic infections. After an initial infection, usually in the mucous membranes of the mouth or anal and genital areas, these viruses remain latent in nerve cells. Infections with these organisms tend to activate cells that have HIV proviruses in their DNA. This activation makes these cells produce more HIV. Infections with herpes simplex virus and *M. tuberculosis* make cells produce more co-receptors (upregulation), making many more cells much more likely to be invaded by HIV. When people with HIV infection have these other infections, HIV disease advances more quickly. They have higher levels of HIV in their blood and transmit HIV much more readily.

On the other hand, HIV-related immunosuppression allows other infections to progress to very severe disease. In most people without HIV infection, warts caused by human papillomaviruses, and genital herpes, fever blisters in the mouth, or shingles caused by herpes viruses occasionally reoccur. People with HIV who are infected with these viruses, however, are plagued with severe, frequent recurrences. These become harder to control as immunosuppression worsens. Often, children and adults with HIV become covered with skin warts for years and may have scarring, painful shingles on their torsos or limbs, or suffer from severe, chronic oral or genital blisters and sores.

Vaginal and oral candidiasis (referred to as "yeast infections" and "thrush") are usually mild infections that annoy but do not endanger women and infants with normal immune systems. In people with HIV, these infections cause stubborn, peeling skin lesions; burning, painful vaginal lesions; and oral lesions that spread into the esophagus, making eating difficult.

Gonorrhea and *Chlamydia trachomatis* are sexually transmitted infections that often cause no symptoms in women, although if untreated, they can cause irreversible damage. In women with HIV, however, these infections quickly rise from the cervix to the womb, the ovaries, and fallopian tubes, causing painful, pus-filled lesions called **tubo-ovarian abscesses**.

A person who does not have HIV but has been infected by these other organisms is more likely to become infected with HIV if exposed to it. Weaknesses in the body's first line of defense against HIV infection (the mucous membranes or skin of the genitals), caused by genital ulcers due to syphilis, genital herpes, or chancroid (a sexually transmitted ulcer), greatly increase the risk that an exposure to HIV will result in HIV transmission. Infections with *Chlamydia trachomatis, Neisseria gonorrhoeae, Trichomonas vaginalis,* and genital infections that are not sexually transmitted, such as bacterial vaginosis and yeast infections, also increase the likelihood that a sexual exposure will result in HIV transmission.

Through different mechanisms, these infections make the uninfected partner more susceptible to infection. Ulcers and infections that cause itching and scratching do this by stripping away protective layers of cells. These and other infections may also cause inflammation, which brings CD4+ T cells to the area that can readily be infected by HIV. Bacterial vaginosis causes the beneficial bacteria that make acid products that protect against HIV to be replaced by other bacteria, which promotes HIV invasion.

5

Diagnosing HIV Infection and AIDS

Soon after the virus that came to be known as HIV was discovered, researchers showed that the virus could be cultured from the blood and lymph nodes of people with the full and varied spectrum of the disease that is known as AIDS. The development of a test that detected antibody to HIV led to a much greater understanding of the natural history of HIV infection. Tests for antibody to HIV have evolved tremendously over the years and have become much better, with fewer false positives and false negatives. Antibody tests can be performed using saliva, blood, or urine.

TESTING FOR HIV ANTIBODY

Although they have evolved considerably, antibody tests for HIV are still based on the strategy that was used in 1985 for HIV diagnosis: an **enzyme-linked immunosorbent assay (ELISA)**. With the most rapid form of this test, a result can be available in 20 to 30 minutes. If the ELISA test is positive twice, a Western blot test is performed to further verify the results. In this test, individual proteins of HIV are separated according to size. The viral proteins are then transferred onto nitrocellulose paper and the patient's serum is added. Any antibody in the patient's serum to each specific HIV protein is detected by an antibody to human antibody (antihuman immunoglobulin G [IgG])

(continued on page 86)

GETTING TESTED FOR HIV

The test for antibody to HIV (HIVab) is one of the most commonly used tests in the world. It is performed using a technique called enzyme-linked immunosorbent assay (ELISA, for short). HIV ELISAs are performed using a clear plastic plate with many wells that have HIV antigen attached to the wells. HIV antigen is protein from HIV that is recognized by HIVab (Figure 5.1).

In the first step, several drops of the part of the blood that has antibodies (serum) from patients who want to be tested are placed into each well. Almost 20 patients can be tested using one plate. If the sample has antibody to HIV, the HIVab will stick to the HIV antigen.

In the second step, another liquid will be placed in each well, and mixed with the serum. This liquid contains antibody to HIVab. This antibody, which has an enzyme attached to it, will find HIVab and latch on to the antibody. At this point, the wells with serum from patients who have HIVab will contain the HIV antigen attached to the well, the patient's HIVab bound to it, and the test kit's antibody to HIVab, which is linked to an enzyme. In the wells with serum from patients without HIVab (not infected), there will be no HIVab. The test kit's antibody to HIVab, along with the enzyme, will just be floating around, and the HIV antigen will be attached to the well, without any connection to the test kit's antibody for the enzyme.

In the third step, all the wells are rinsed. In wells that do not contain HIVab, the antibody to HIVab with enzyme is washed off. However, if the antibody to HIVab is present, the antibody to HIVab and the enzyme will not wash off; it will stay bound to HIVab.

In the last step, a chemical is added that, in the presence of the enzyme, turns a bright yellow color. If there is enzyme in the well (attached to the antibody to HIVab, which in turn is attached to the HIVab and the HIV antigen in the

GETTING TESTED FOR HIV *(continued)*

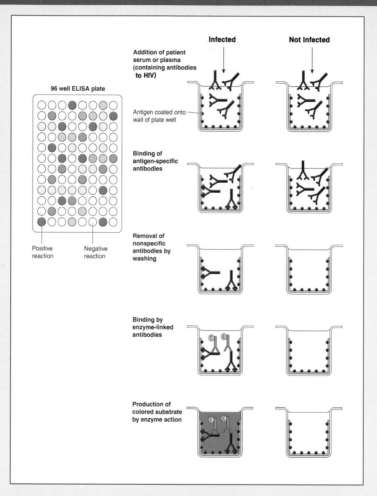

Figure 5.1 The enzyme-linked immunosorbent assay (ELISA) to detect antibody to HIV is illustrated here. Serum from a test subject is added to a microwell coated with HIV antigens. If the HIV antibody is present in the test serum, it will bind to the HIV antigens already in the well. The wells are then rinsed, and any serum that did not have HIV antibody (and thus did not bind to the antigen) will be washed away. Then, antibodies that bind only to HIV-antibodies and have an enzyme linked to them are added to the wells. A substrate is added that will only change color if HIV antibody is present in the well, denoting a positive response (infected).

well), it will catalyze a reaction (make the reaction proceed) and turn the liquid in the well bright yellow. This means that the sample contains HIVab (a "positive" reaction). If there is no enzyme in the well (because there is no HIVab), the sample remains clear, and the sample is considered negative. Samples that yield a positive result are repeated.

If the sample is again positive, another test called a Western blot is performed. It tests for antibodies to several HIV antigens that are stuck on a thin strip of material called nitrocellulose. The serum is added to the strip, and the strip is placed in a special instrument that runs an electric current through the nitrocellulose. If a dark stripe (or "band") forms where the HIV antigens were placed, the test is said to be positive (Figure 5.2).

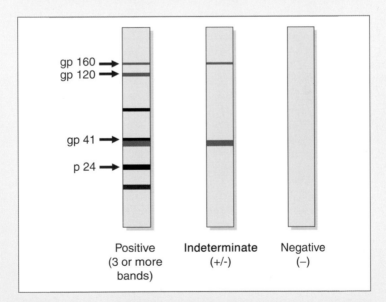

Figure 5.2 If a serum sample yields a positive response to the ELISA test twice, a more specific test called a Western blot is performed. In this test, antibodies to three or more HIV antigens (glycoproteins 160, 120, or 41, designated as "gp") or protein (designated as "p") 24 have to be present in the sample for the test to be positive. Glycoproteins and proteins are named for their molecular weights.

(continued from page 82)

mixed with an enzyme that, in the presence of human antibody, makes a colored band.

If no bands are visible, the Western blot is said to be negative. Even if the ELISA test is positive two or more times, the HIV antibody test is said to be negative if there are no bands at all in the Western blot test. If there are bands, showing that there is antibody to protein 24 and to glycoprotein 41, generally only seen among people with HIV infection, the test is positive. If there are bands in any other combination, the test is called indeterminate (meaning that it is not possible to determine whether the results are positive or negative).

If the Western blot test from a blood donor has any bands at all, the blood donation is not used. People whose tests are indeterminate are encouraged to have repeat testing, since at least some of them will actually turn out not to be infected.

When a person is infected with HIV, there is a window of time in which there is no detectable antibody in the blood. Even some people who are truly infected have negative HIV tests early in the course of infection. The newest HIV antibody tests can detect antibody fairly soon after infection with HIV (within one to three months).

Testing for HIV in Babies

Even if a mother is untreated, less than 50% of infants born to women with HIV are infected by mother-to-child transmission. However, most infants born to women with HIV infection have antibody to HIV. That is because the placenta allows the passage of antibodies from the mother to the baby to protect the baby from many infectious diseases to which the mother is immune. Along with all the other antibodies, HIV antibody will also reach the baby through the placenta. As a result, the HIV antibody tests cannot be used to diagnose HIV in the baby for months, until the antibody from the mother is no longer present.

TESTING FOR THE VIRUS AND FOR IMMUNE FUNCTION

Tests that detect the virus itself (not just the antibody to the virus) must be used to diagnose HIV infection in babies or in older children and adults before HIV antibody is present, and to see whether HIV is already affecting immune function. These tests consist of:

- Polymerase chain reaction tests;

- CD4 or T cell counts.

Polymerase Chain Reaction Tests

Polymerase chain reaction tests are performed by collecting blood from the patient, using an enzyme that finds fragments of HIV RNA or DNA-provirus in the patient's blood, and using polymerase (an enzyme) to catalyze a reaction that multiplies the nucleic acid by thousands to millions of times in the laboratory. The enzyme, polymerase, makes many copies of the nucleic acid. This allows the magnified nucleic acid to be easily detected. Polymerase tests can determine not only that there is HIV in the blood, but also how many HIV particles are in each milliliter of blood. High counts of virus are seen usually when HIV infection is progressing. Much lower or undetectable levels are seen usually during the early phase of infection or when the person is responding well to antiretrovirals.

Although viral counts of HIV are very useful, they have some limitations. For unclear reasons, low counts are not as reliable in women as they are in men. Virtually all men with low viral counts do not have severe disease or are responding to treatment. However, even women who have very severe HIV disease or are dying sometimes have low viral counts.

CD4 or T Cell Counts

The number of CD4+ T cells per milliliter, sometimes called the CD4 or T cell count, is a more reliable test of a patient's extent of immunosuppression than the viral loads. This test is performed using flow cytometry. Flow cytometry sorts cells in blood based on physical and other traits (Figure 5.3). Flow cytometry allows a single cell from a blood sample to be checked for several characteristics as it flows in liquid past a light source. The cells scatter or absorb light, and flow cytometers measure the light that the cells emit.

THE "CD4 COUNT"

In the 1980s, soon after HIV was discovered, scientists noticed that HIV had a special liking for helper T cells. Some scientists thought that the cluster designation (CD) 4 molecule (which only helper T cells have) acted as a "handle" for HIV to hook onto a helper T cell and infect it. In experiments, scientists could "block" the CD4 molecule by mixing antibodies with CD4. Then, HIV could not bind to the helper cell and could not infect it. They suspected that maybe the CD4 molecule itself was a receptor for HIV. Maybe HIV needed to stick to the CD4 molecule to be able to infect the helper cell.

Drs. Steve McDougal and Janine Jason have special training in immunology. Before AIDS was first recognized, Dr. Jason wrote an article about what was known about how helper T cells worked. During the early 1980s, both doctors did very important work on HIV, studying how HIV was being spread to people with hemophilia, and how it could be stopped.

The first case of AIDS in a hemophiliac was discovered in 1981, just a few months after the very first *Morbidity and Mortality Weekly Report* article. But it took a lot of hard work by Drs. McDougal, Jason, and others to convince the public (particularly blood banks) that blood products were spreading the disease. Other studies showed how the number of helper T cells decreased as HIV infection progressed.

In 1986, Dr. McDougal and other CDC scientists performed an experiment. They took helper T cells and put radioactive "labels" on them. Then, they added HIV to the

To determine the number of CD4+ T cells, antibodies to CD4 are attached to a fluorescent green dye. Antibodies to CD8 are attached to a fluorescent red dye. Both of these antibodies are then mixed with the T cells from a patient. The antibodies that have the green dye bind tightly to CD4. During flow cytometry, T cells that have CD4 glow bright green. T cells that have CD8 glow red. T cells that have both CD4

cells. HIV antibodies bound to a cell surface protein. The protein (CD4) was identified through other experiments. Two antibodies to CD4 were tested to see if they could bind with the CD4 molecule when HIV was present. When HIV was bound to the CD4, it blocked the binding of one of the antibodies, but not the other. When HIV was "labeled" and stuck to helper T cells, a viral glycoprotein (gp) weighing 110 kilodaltons (gp110) stuck to the CD4 molecule. The gp110 appeared to be a major factor in infection! During the first 18 months after this article was published, other scientists cited it in their own research more than 120 times.

Gp110 turned out not to be as important to making medicines and vaccines to fight HIV as was first hoped. It is now known that there are other receptors in addition to CD4 that are important for HIV infection to occur. However, the count of how many CD4+ T cells a patient has per cubic milliliter or, as it is often called, the "CD4 count" remains a very important way of checking the prognosis of people with HIV. Dr. McDougal's experiments were critical in understanding how HIV affects helper T cells. Some version of his experiments is part of much of the research to test HIV vaccines and treatments. His work on how heat and chemicals affect HIV has made treating hemophilia with blood products much safer for patients. Doctors McDougal, Jason, and many others working on the effects of HIV infection in the 1980s and 1990s learned a lot about how the cell-mediated immune system works.

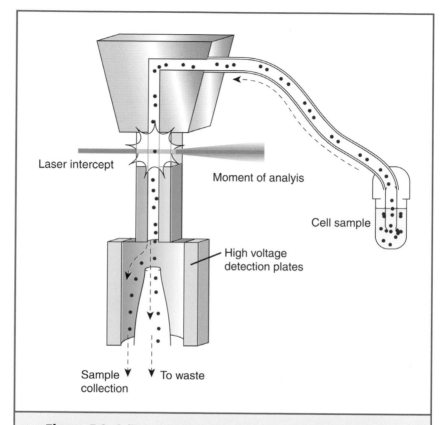

Laser intercept

Moment of analyis

Cell sample

High voltage
detection plates

Sample ▼ ▼ To waste
collection

Figure 5.3 A flow cytometer, illustrated here, counts the number of T cells that are CD4+ ("helper") cells and the number that are CD8 ("suppressor") cells, by detecting whether they emit green or red light. Flow cytometry can also be used to differentiate other cells based on their characteristics.

and CD8 emit both green and red light. This information gives a measure of how many of each type of T cell were present in the blood specimen and is turned into a two-dimensional image digitally.

Normally, infants and young children have over 1,000 CD4+ T cells per cubic milliliter of blood. They may show signs of immune suppression even with 500 or more CD4+ T cells per cubic milliliter. Adults normally have lower numbers of these

T cells and rarely have immune suppression when their CD4+ T cell count is above 200. In most people, regardless of age, when the proportion of lymphocytes that are CD4+ falls below 25%, signs of immune suppression soon follow. For that reason, doctors sometimes prefer to follow the percentage of lymphocytes that are CD4+, instead of the absolute numbers. In this way, they can check progress of immune suppression or response to medicine for years, even in babies and young children, using the same ruler.

6

Treating HIV Infection With Antiretroviral Drugs

ANTIRETROVIRAL DRUGS

Antiretroviral drugs work by inhibiting some viral activities. The three major drug classes are:

- Reverse transcriptase inhibitors;

- Protease inhibitors;

- Fusion inhibitors.

The different classes of medicines, and the medicines in each class, have different ways of inhibiting viral attacks without harming the human patient. As described in this chapter, each of these types of drugs is effective at different points of the HIV life cycle (see Figure 6.1). However, all of these drugs can have serious side effects, some of which can be fatal. Some side effects are specific for each drug; other side effects are caused by virtually all of the drugs. Most patients with HIV infection who need antiretrovirals find a combination of drugs that they can tolerate. However, some patients cannot tolerate any antiretroviral drugs due to side effects.

Reverse Transcriptase Inhibitors

The first generation of antiretroviral medicine consisted of nucleoside

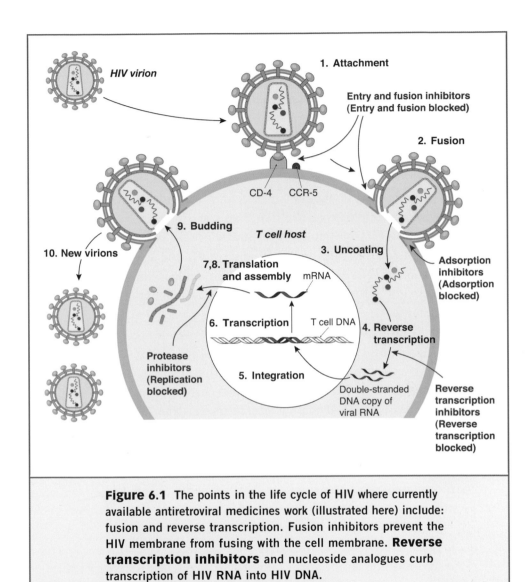

Figure 6.1 The points in the life cycle of HIV where currently available antiretroviral medicines work (illustrated here) include: fusion and reverse transcription. Fusion inhibitors prevent the HIV membrane from fusing with the cell membrane. **Reverse transcription inhibitors** and nucleoside analogues curb transcription of HIV RNA into HIV DNA.

analogues (or imitation nucleosides). They look almost like real nucleosides, the chemicals that make the "steps" in the ladder-like DNA molecule. Reverse trancriptase picks up these analogues as if they were real nucleosides, not noticing the subtle difference, and then attaches them to the proviral

DNA chain that it is making to put into the nucleus. The nucleoside analogue does not have a place for another "link" to be added, and reverse transcriptase cannot add more nucleoside links to the nucleic acid chain. The DNA chain ends at this point, and the production of HIV DNA is halted.

Because they block reverse transcriptase activity, these antiretroviral medicines are called **reverse transcriptase inhibitors (RTIs)**. RTIs that are analogues for nucleosides (e.g., adenosine, thymidine) are called **nucleoside reverse transcriptase inhibitors (NRTIs)**. This class includes zidovudine (AZT), lamivudine (3TC), stavudine (d4T), abacavir (ABC), didanosine (ddI), dideoxycitidine (ddC), and tenofovir. The approved combinations of NRTIs are Combivir® (a combination of AZT and 3TC) and Trizivir® (a combination of abacavir, AZT, and 3TC). Combivir and Trizivir come as pills that are taken one in the morning and one at night.

Some antiretroviral drugs are not analogues of nucleosides, but they still inhibit reverse transcriptase by attaching to the reverse transcriptase enzyme and curbing its action. These drugs are called **non-nucleoside reverse transcriptase inhibitors (NNRTIs)** and include Efavirenz, Nevirapine, and Delavirdine. This class of drugs is popular with many patients because they only have to be taken once a day. A commonly used combination is two NRTIs (like Combivir) and one NNRTI (usually Efavirenz).

A disadvantage of Efavirenz is that it makes birth control pills less effective and it can cause severe birth defects, mostly related to failure of the spinal cord of the baby to fuse during gestation. When the baby is born, parts of the spinal cord are still outside of the body, and the nerve tissue below that part of the body may be damaged, causing the child to be unable to move its legs or to control the bladder and bowels.

The disadvantage of Nevirapine is that it sometimes causes liver side effects, including severe, permanent liver failure necessitating a liver transplant, or even death.

Tenofovir is a drug in the last class of reverse transcriptase inhibitors—nucleotide analogue RTIs. The only difference between how nucleoside analogues and this nucleotide analogue work is that the nucleoside analogues have to be activated in the body to actually reverse transcriptase. Tenofovir is already activated when it enters the body.

Protease Inhibitors

Protease inhibitors (PIs) block the ability of protease enzymes to clip the long strands of amino acids into working proteins for HIV. Used in combination with RTIs, protease inhibitors are the strongest anti-HIV treatment available today; 90% of patients who take combination antiretrovirals that include protease inhibitors respond to the treatment. This response lasts many months, even years.

Combinations of reverse transcriptase and protease inhibitors are synergistic; together, they work far better than one would think from adding their separate antiretroviral effects. Using protease inhibitors with reverse transcriptase inhibitors also greatly decreases the chance that viruses resistant to any antiretroviral medicine will emerge.

The disadvantages of protease inhibitors, however, are many. Most protease inhibitors do not mix well with water. Some have to be taken on an empty stomach. Others can only be taken with low-fat meals. They are broken down very quickly in the body, so they must be taken three or more times a day. These characteristics make them more complicated to use than the reverse transcriptase inhibitors, which can be taken once or twice a day and with any kind of food. They are also more expensive than the reverse transcriptase inhibitors. In addition, they have even more unwanted interactions with other medicines.

Although most antiretrovirals can cause abnormalities in how the body processes and stores fats, the protease inhibitors

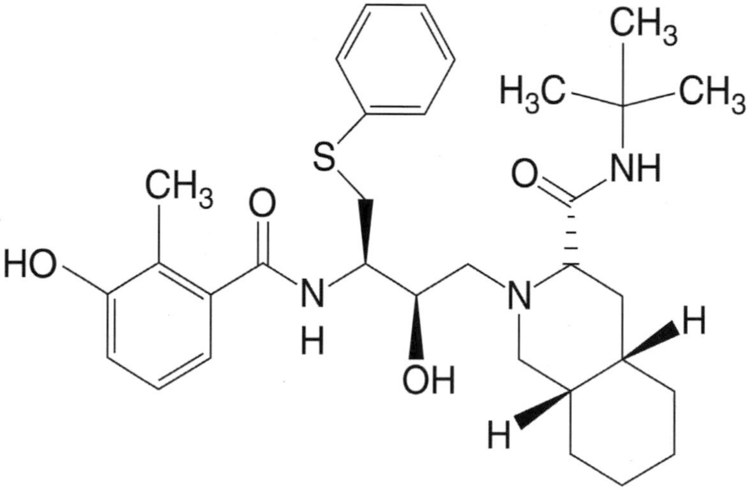

Figure 6.2 Nelfinavir (shown here) and the other protease inhibitors, which are, to date, the most effective antiretroviral drugs, are not naturally occurring chemicals. Researchers designed these medicines based on the structure of the protease enzyme, targeting its active site. HIV protease cuts large inactive virus proteins ("polyproteins") into essential working proteins (including reverse transcriptase, p24, and integrase) as each new virion buds from an HIV-infected cell. The genetically engineered protease inhibitors fit perfectly into the protease, lock it up, and shut it down so polyproteins are not cut. The virus cannot mature, bud, and infect a new cell.

are much more likely to cause these effects. Among these side effects is lipodystrophy, which includes loss of fat in the face and buttocks and increased fat between the shoulder blades and in the abdomen.

Protease inhibitors currently available are Saquivanir, Ritonavir, Indinavir, Lopinavir, and Nelfinavir (Figure 6.2). Kaletra® is the brand name of a combination of Lopinavir and Ritonavir. Ritonavir inhibits an enzyme that breaks down Lopinavir, so there is a lot more Lopinavir in the body when it is combined with Ritonavir. Thus, Kaletra makes a smaller amount of Lopinavir go a much longer way than it would alone, reducing the side effects related to protease inhibitors while increasing effectiveness.

Fusion Inhibitors

In March 2003, the FDA approved the first of a new class of antiretrovirals: **fusion inhibitors**. The fusion inhibitor, called enfuvirtide (T-20), binds glycoprotein (GP)41, a chemical in the virus membrane, and acts against it.

When HIV first attaches to a cell, two regions of GP41 mix with each other in a kind of molecular shape change. This allows the membranes to stick together so that HIV can inject its DNA into the cell. T-20 probably acts by preventing this GP41 change, thus blocking fusion entirely. The approved drug can only be taken by injection, not by mouth. Its use gives hope to those patients who no longer respond to other antiretroviral drugs.

RESISTANCE TO ANTIRETROVIRALS

HIV develops **resistance** to antiretrovirals quickly. Generally, when HIV becomes resistant to one medicine in a drug class, it will have some resistance to other members of that drug class.

A virus is resistant to a drug when the antiretrovirals no longer harm the virus. This resistance occurs because the virus multiplies very fast, yielding **mutants** of the virus. Some mutants may be resistant to the antiretroviral. The antiretroviral drug will kill viruses that are not resistant, allowing a type of **natural selection** to occur. Only the virus that is resistant to the drug will survive; it can then reproduce without any competition. Soon, millions, then billions, of resistant virus particles take over.

To delay the time when most of a patient's virus particles are resistant to the drugs, combinations of drugs are used. Combinations make it harder for the virus to become resistant.

Viruses need to have several mutations in the same organism to become resistant to several antiretrovirals at a time. Eventually, however, most viruses in a patient will become resistant to drugs. For this reason, it is best not to start the patient on antiretroviral drugs until they are really needed. Then, it is essential to start with a combination of drugs that will kill HIV most effectively. That way, the number of reproducing viruses from which resistant mutants can spring will stay low. Recently, scientists have seen that some resistant mutants are not as dangerous to the patient as the nonresistant, naturally occuring "wild-type" HIV. Patients appear not to be responding to treatment. Their viral loads are high, and tests on their HIV show that they are very resistant. Yet when the treatment is discontinued, and the "wild-type" nonresistant HIV takes over, the patients get much sicker, with symptoms and signs of severe immunosuppression.

HIGHLY ACTIVE ANTIRETROVIRAL THERAPY

Highly active antiretroviral therapy (HAART) consists of a combination of at least three antiretroviral drugs. No antiretroviral drugs work well alone once a person is infected. How faithfully a patient continues to take the medicines is very important, since it is crucial to keep a high enough level of antiretrovirals in the system so partially resistant mutants cannot be selected for survival.

When a person is diagnosed with HIV, he or she should undergo a physical examination and laboratory tests. Blood tests are performed to see how the liver and kidneys are functioning, how many CD4+ T cells are present, and if enough red blood cells are being made.

Currently, most physicians specializing in the treatment of HIV believe that it is best to let the patient's defenses fight the virus until the T cell numbers drop, indicating that the body is not able to fight infection normally. Once the number of CD4+ T cells in each milliliter drops below 350, most HIV specialists recommend starting HAART. Also, if the patient develops an opportunistic infection or if the level of virus in the blood is very high, many doctors suggest starting HAART.

SIDE EFFECTS

Antiretroviral drugs differ from each other in many ways, especially the side effects they cause. Some combinations of drugs work better than others. Certain antiretrovirals reduce the effectiveness of other antiretrovirals. Some side effects of common antiretrovirals are listed in Table 6.1.

SIDE EFFECTS AND INTERACTIONS OF ANTIRETROVIRALS

Most medicines, even common medications such as penicillin and aspirin, have side effects. Some medicines interact in a negative way with other medications. They can decrease the effectiveness of other medicines, increase the side effects of other medications, or be weakened or made more toxic by other medications. It is important to note that antiretrovirals have many side effects, some of which lead to permanent organ damage. They also have many interactions with medicines that people with HIV tend to need.

It is a good rule of thumb to avoid medications unless they are needed. However, this rule is particularly important with antiretrovirals. In general, the more severe immuno-suppression is at the start of antiretroviral treatment, and the more other medicines the patient needs, the more likely that a serious side effect or interaction will occur. Women are particularly likely to have serious side effects involving the liver due to various medicines when they are pregnant. The medicine may also harm the baby. Some antiretrovirals can cause birth defects, so they are avoided in the treatment of pregnant women with HIV if there is another antiretroviral that can be used instead.

Table 6.1: Side Effects of Commonly Used Antiretroviral Medications

DRUG	SIDE EFFECT
NUCLEOSIDE REVERSE TRANSCRIPTASE INHIBITORS	
Zidovudine (AZT)	Decrease in granulocytes, decrease in red blood cells (anemia)
Didanosine (ddI)	Inflammation of the pancreas, damage to nerves of the hands and feet, diarrhea, liver damage
Zalcitabine (ddC)	Inflammation of the pancreas, vomiting, damage to nerves of the hands and feet, rash, sores in the mouth
Stavudine (d4T)	Inflammation of the pancreas, damage to nerves of the hands and feet, severe liver damage (particularly in pregnant women), decrease in red blood cells (anemia), headache, insomnia
Lamivudine (3TC)	Inflammation of the pancreas, damage to nerves of the hands and feet, rash, cough, dizziness, fatigue, stomachache, headache, insomnia, hair loss
NUCLEOTIDE ANALOGUE REVERSE TRANSCRIPTASE INHIBITORS	
Tenofovir	Nausea, vomiting, diarrhea, gas, decreased bone mineral levels, kidney damage
NON-NUCLEOSIDE REVERSE TRANSCRIPTASE INHIBITORS	
Nevirapine	Rash, fever, headaches, nausea, mouth ulcers, rare but very severe or fatal liver damage
Efavirenz	Dizziness, nightmares, hallucinations, confusion and psychiatric disturbances; if taken during first weeks of pregnancy, can cause birth defect of the baby's spinal cord
PROTEASE INHIBITORS	
Saquinavir	Diarrhea, stomachache, nausea, rash
Ritonavir	Nausea, vomiting, diarrhea, fatigue, abnormal sensation around the mouth, headache, sugar diabetes
Indinavir	Kidney damage, jaundice, stomachache, fatigue, flank pain, nausea, vomiting, diarrhea, heartburn, back pain, headache, insomnia, dizziness, sugar diabetes
Nelfinavir	Diarrhea, rash, headache, nausea, sugar diabetes
FUSION INHIBITORS	
Enfuvirtide	Headache, dizziness, insomnia, muscle aches, damage to nerves of the hands and feet

Reverse transcriptase inhibitors curb HIV transcription thousands of times more than the normal transcription that human cells need. But they do affect normal human cells to some degree. They can greatly reduce the ability of the bone marrow to make red blood cells, which normally need to be replaced constantly. This results in anemia. In some people, this anemia can be easily controlled with other medications. Others, however, cannot tolerate the anemia.

Some antiretrovirals cause liver damage, but many people with HIV infection can actually tolerate medicines that cause some liver damage without compromising important liver functions. However, people whose liver is already damaged from hepatitis B or C, diseases that are often spread among injection drug users or result from chronic alcohol abuse, may not be able to tolerate even minimal further liver damage.

7

Preventing HIV Infection and AIDS

In industrialized countries during the 20th century, the number of deaths caused by infectious diseases decreased dramatically. For example, as the 1900s dawned, syphilis was an incurable disease and a major cause of death. But many measures to prevent syphilis and to prevent the worst outcomes in those who acquired syphilis were introduced and helped reduce the number of cases, even before penicillin was discovered as a treatment. Because the microorganisms that cause syphilis and HIV are spread in a similar way, some of the methods successfully used to prevent the spread of syphilis, including screening, helping infected people inform their sex partners that they need to be tested, and showing people how to protect themselves, also work well to prevent the spread of HIV.

REDUCING THE SPREAD OF HIV

Very early in the course of the HIV pandemic, researchers recognized the importance of prevention. In 1988, every household in the United States received a letter from the Surgeon General informing them of the need to take specific measures to prevent the spread of HIV (Figure 7.1). Because most people who were infected did not know they were infected, people were encouraged to assume, unless they knew otherwise, that any sex partner might be infected. Other preventive measures included encouraging adolescents and young adults to delay sexual activity and encouraging the use of condoms during sex. Because of some anatomic characteristics of the adolescent sex organs, adolescent girls are much more likely to get infected if exposed to HIV than are adult women or men who have sex

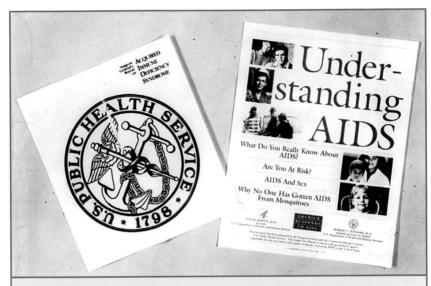

Figure 7.1 In 1988, then Surgeon General Dr. C. Everett Koop sent a pamphlet entitled "Understanding AIDS" to every household in the United States to alert Americans about the HIV threat. The pamphlet, shown here, outlined some of the facts and myths about the disease, as well as risk factors.

only with women. During adolescence, almost half of young women have temporary migration of cells inside the cervix (mouth of the womb) to the outside of the womb and into the vagina. These cells are much more vulnerable to HIV than the cells that normally cover the cervix. Delaying sex into adulthood is likely to reduce the risk of HIV for young women.

In the years since that first letter was sent, researchers, community-based advocates, and government scientists have worked with the print and broadcast media to encourage prevention strategies, which have been extremely effective. During the 1990s, dramatic decreases in the number of adolescents who had had sex and marked increases in the number who used condoms if they did have sex were seen. The estimated number of new HIV infections decreased by almost half, in large part due to these behavioral changes.

Reducing Sexual Transmission

Most HIV transmission in the United States, as worldwide, occurs from sexual contact. Even small reductions in the risk of sexual HIV transmission can greatly reduce the number of new cases of HIV. The most effective measure to prevent sexual transmission of HIV is for uninfected people not to engage in any sexual activities with people who have HIV infection. Ways to accomplish this include:

- **Abstinence**—not engaging in sexual activities that can transmit HIV

- **Monogamy**—engaging in sexual activities only with one person, who is also uninfected.

Not every sex act between a person with HIV and an uninfected partner results in HIV transmission. Many factors greatly increase the risk that an exposure will result in transmission. Among these are infections or irritation of the sexual organs, often caused by sexually transmitted diseases such as herpes and syphilis, and non-sexually transmitted infections such as yeast infections. In groups where HIV infection is not very common, reducing the number of sex partners can greatly decrease the risk of inadvertently having sex with an infected person.

Trauma to the sex organs during sex also greatly increases the risk of HIV transmission. Therefore, preventing trauma during sex with lubrication and avoiding sexual activities that result in scratches or bleeding reduce risk. Getting appropriate treatment for STDs and other infections of the genitals also greatly decreases the risk of HIV transmission. So can an individual's decision to avoid products that increase the risk of HIV transmission, such as **douches** and **spermicides** containing nonoxynol-9. Nonoxynol-9, the spermicide found in all birth control vaginal creams and jellies in the United States, was tested to see if it prevented HIV infection. It was found not to

(continued on page 107)

WHERE THE RUBBER HITS THE ROAD

During the first epidemiologic studies of AIDS in the early 1980s, researchers noted that people who used male latex **condoms** (in heterosexual or male/male sexual interactions) seemed to be at far lower risk of developing the disease. Previously, latex condoms had been used mainly to prevent pregnancy and the spread of several sexually transmitted infections, for which they were quite effective. Condoms were studied very intensely to determine their effectiveness in preventing the spread of HIV.

These studies were not like the randomized clinical trials to test medicines and other products, because it would be unthinkable to assign someone to a damaged or "placebo" condom. The studies were "observational." They looked at couples where one person was infected with HIV, and people who were often sexually exposed to others who had HIV. Except for a tiny fraction of people who, for some reason, remained uninfected (individuals who are highly exposed, persistently sero-negative [HEPS]; see Chapter 4), many, if not most, people who reportedly had unprotected sex with infected partners became infected.

However, if the male partner in the relationship used a male latex condom correctly each and every time that there was vaginal or anal intercourse, whether he was the infected partner or not, the risk of acquiring or spreading HIV dramatically decreased. This was true despite the fact that HIV is much smaller than a sperm cell or one of the sexually transmitted bacteria. The difference in risk of HIV infection among condom users compared to condom nonusers was much more dramatic than the difference in risk of pregnancy or sexually transmitted bacterial disease among condom users compared to nonusers. This may be because the number of HIV particles needed to spread the infection by sex is much higher than the number of sperm cells needed to ensure pregnancy. It is also greater than the number of microorganisms needed to spread gonorrhea, for example.

WHERE THE RUBBER HITS THE ROAD (continued)

According to this and similar studies, the protective effect of using male latex condoms (Figure 7.2) correctly and consistently, if there is no slipping or tearing, is higher than 85%, and may exceed 90%. Condom effectiveness depends on using a condom each and every time there is intercourse. This is sometimes not very easy. For the foreseeable future, even if microbicides and vaccines are developed, male latex condoms remain the most effective protection against HIV for sexually active people who are not in a monogamous relationship with an uninfected partner.

Fewer than half of adults in the United States, and a low percentage of adults worldwide, have been tested for HIV. It is estimated that about 25% of people who are living with HIV in the United States do not know that they have HIV infection. Most people who discover they have HIV infection take steps to reduce the likelihood that they will spread HIV to others. However, people who do not know their HIV status, or those who know that they are infected but do not act on this information, are the source of thousands of new infections each year. In addition, a negative antibody test gives a great deal of assurance, but not a 100% guarantee, that a person is not infected. Therefore, it is vitally important that people reduce their risk of HIV infection if they engage in any activities that can transmit HIV with partners whose infection status is unknown.

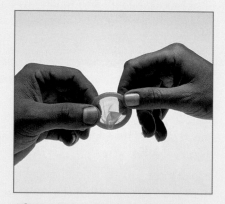

Figure 7.2 Condoms are a very effective way to prevent pregnancy and many sexually transmitted diseases, such as HIV. Male rubber latex condoms are packaged rolled into a doughnut shape and are available for a low cost.

(continued from page 104)

be effective, and, in fact, in some cases, may actually increase risk of HIV infection, probably because it causes irritation and microscopic sores in vaginal mucous membranes. These products also kill normal bacteria that protect the vagina from HIV infection. Anal intercourse is far more likely to result in transmission if either partner is infected; unprotected anal intercourse with partners who are infected is very likely to result in spread of HIV.

Using Condoms to Prevent HIV Transmission

Male condoms are extremely effective in preventing the transmission of HIV. However, they are not a foolproof solution. Some men, particularly beginners, have a difficult time having sex if they use them. If the insertive partner cannot or will not use condoms correctly and consistently, the receptive partner cannot protect him or herself.

Receptive partners have expressed their need for prevention methods that they can control themselves. A tremendous research effort is under way to find ways to assist receptive partners, particularly women, to reduce their risk of HIV infection during sex (see Chapter 8). Female condoms were developed to respond to these needs. Even ways of helping uninfected female partners of men with HIV conceive and give birth to babies without contracting HIV infection are being explored.

Reducing Exposure From Injection Drug Use

Using needles or syringes to inject drugs that may have been used before by someone with HIV is very likely to result in transmission of HIV to the next user. Considerable effort has been directed at reducing HIV transmission due to injection drug use. Providing people who are dependent on injected substances with rehabilitation has been very effective in reducing their risk of HIV and many other infections, including hepatitis B and C.

For others who continue injecting, needle-exchange programs are a very promising solution. Many injection drug users reuse needles because antidrug laws make it illegal for them to obtain or even possess injection equipment. Needle-exchange programs supply sterile needles for injection drug users so they do not have to share or reuse their injection equipment.

HE SAID, SHE SAID: THE FEMALE CONDOM

As of 1989, there was a lot of information available to convince the FDA that use of the male latex condom decreased the risk of HIV infection. However, male latex condoms had some problems. There are some people who are allergic to latex rubber. Some people complained that their partners could not or would not use latex condoms because they slightly decreased sensation. Latex condoms can only be used with water-based lubricants, like K-Y® Jelly, as oils or Vaseline® weakens them. Most importantly, the use of male latex condoms is something that only the male inserting partner really controls. Women wanted a method that they could use themselves.

A lot of research went into designing a "condom" that a woman could insert into the vagina for protection. The result of this research was the female condom, a sheath made out of polyurethane, a very thin but very strong plastic. It has a "blind" end that is inserted in the vagina and fits over the mouth of the womb, held in place by a small plastic ring. The other end has a larger ring, and is open. This ring stays outside of the vagina (Figure 7.3). The woman places the blind end inside her vagina up to eight hours before intercourse.

Studies performed in the early 1990s showed that the female condom was about as effective as the male condom in decreasing the risk of pregnancy and sexually transmitted diseases. The female condom has some problems, however. Although any type of lubricant can be used, a lot of lubrication is needed. Otherwise, the condom makes a lot of noise. Some people think it does not look as "nice" as the male condom. It is also more than twice as expensive as a male condom, but can

Needle-exchange programs are very effective, but they are also also very controversial. Some people think these programs decrease the motivation of substance-dependent people to seek rehabilitation. Others suggest that for many injection drug users,

only be used once, just like the male condom. It takes some training and practice to use. The female condom really cannot be used without the male partner's cooperation. It is obvious that it is there, since it is hanging out of the woman's vagina. One or both partners sometimes feel discomfort during its use.

Many men, however, like the female condom, or at least do not mind it. Because the material is much thinner, and less tight than a male condom, some men feel it is more comfortable. Studies have shown that people that have both male and female condoms available are much less likely to have sex acts that are unprotected than people who have just male condoms. The FDA approved the female condom in 1993. It has become, with the male condom, an important tool for decreasing risk of pregnancy and STDs, particularly HIV, for sexually active people who may not be in monogamous relationships with uninfected partners.

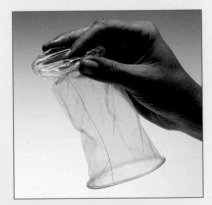

Figure 7.3 The female condom (shown here) is made of plastic, rather than rubber latex like male condoms. The condoms are larger than male condoms and have a closed end that fits against the cervix. They are more expensive than male condoms.

needle exchange is their first contact with prevention issues, and their first step toward eventually opting for rehabilitation. This type of prevention, which seeks to minimize the harmful effects of high-risk behaviors while trying to also reduce the behaviors themselves, is called **harm reduction.**

Reducing HIV Transmission From Mother to Child

HIV infection acquired by an infant from the mother is the regrettable result of a process that starts before the pregnancy. A woman can dramatically reduce the chance that her child will become infected by:

- Protecting herself from being exposed to HIV infection before and during pregnancy;

- Preventing the pregnancy if she knows she has HIV infection and does not want to have a child;

- Getting treated for HIV during pregnancy and not breast-feeding the baby after it is born, thereby safeguarding her child from the infection during pregnancy, childbirth, and infancy and preventing her child from becoming an orphan.

Women who have HIV infection can take steps to avoid passing the infection on to their babies.

- During the first months of pregnancy, there is very little risk to the baby from contact with the mother's blood. Thus, testing during pregnancy and taking antiretroviral medicines during pregnancy, particularly in the last weeks when almost all HIV transmission takes place, can decrease the risk of mother-to-child transmission to less than 2%.

- If not detected during pregnancy, HIV infection can be detected by testing the mother during labor and delivery.

(continued on page 113)

SPERM WASHING

In the late 1980s, many men with hemophilia learned they had HIV infection. Some wanted to have a child before they died. However, that meant having sex with their wives without a condom. Because not every act of intercourse results in transmission, some tried to pinpoint their wives' most fertile days and only had sex on that day. Of 97 women who used this way of trying to have a baby with their HIV-infected husband, 4 became infected, an unacceptably high number. Semen of men with HIV infection transmits HIV because it contains white blood cells with receptors that HIV can use to get inside other cells. It also has "free" HIV in the liquid portion. But HIV is not believed to be able to infect sperm cells themselves.

In the United States, the first attempts at "sperm washing" included centrifugation (rapid spinning) of semen in a test tube. The sperm cells would settle on the bottom of the tube, while the liquid portion would remain on top. The liquid could then be removed. The sperm cells in the bottom of the tube were then placed in the vaginas or wombs of the uninfected wives of men with HIV. One woman became infected from the procedure, and this experiment was not approved by United States research agencies. In 1990, the CDC and the American Society for Reproductive Medicine (ASRM) strongly cautioned that HIV-discordant (HIV+ male, HIV- female) couples not try to become biological parents.

Far more is now known about how HIV is spread through sex. A researcher in Italy, Dr. Auguste Semprini, and other European researchers, explored ways to decrease the risk of passing HIV from a man to his female partner during the transfer of semen. Thanks to highly active antiretroviral therapy, many men with HIV have lived without symptoms for more than 15 years after finding out that they had HIV. Some have gone years without detectable HIV nucleic acids in their blood. Some men and their wives were willing to let Dr. Semprini try to help them have a child. His "sperm washing" also utilizes centrifugation. However, after the semen fluid is removed, liquid is added to the "pellet" at the bottom of the tube. The sperm cells are then allowed to "swim up" to the surface. The thin layer of fluid with the sperm cells is removed and tested for HIV's RNA using the polymerase chain reaction technique. If there is less HIV nucleic acid than the test can detect, then the sperm are placed in the woman's uterus.

Dr. Semprini's publications suggest that thousands of women have had the procedure and hundreds of babies have been born using this technique and none of the mothers or babies has become infected. HIV is spread to babies from an infected mother, and not from the father. Thus, if the mother is not infected, the baby will not have HIV infection either.

In the United States, several researchers are trying to duplicate Dr. Semprini's methods. In Boston, Dr. Ann Kiessling has proposed to use a procedure similar to Dr. Semprini's. However, for extra safety, she would test all the portions of the semen, even the portions that are rinsed off, not just the sperm. She would not use the sperm if any semen portions have HIV nucleic acid. Then, she would perform in vitro fertilization, taking an egg cell from the mother and mixing it with the sperm cells before placing the fertilized egg into the womb of the mother.

Other U.S. researchers are proposing using the centrifugation and swim up procedure, but placing the sperm at the cervix, not inside the uterus as Dr. Semprini does, to decrease the risk of accidental scratches to the uterus. Others think injecting the sperm after processing into the cytoplasm of the egg, and then putting the fertilized egg in the uterus, would decrease the number of times that couples would need to try before the woman became pregnant. With each time the procedure is attempted, the woman's risk of becoming infected increases.

SPERM WASHING (continued)

There is really no way to guarantee with 100% certainty that the woman will not become infected with HIV. However, researchers have shown success with the sperm washing technique and, based upon the results of Semprini and others, the ASRM is reevaluating its position on sperm washing. Dr. Kiessling and colleagues are gearing up to offer this option to the hundreds of HIV-discordant couples in the United States that are interested in having the procedure.

(continued from page 110)

- Most mother-to-child transmission occurs during delivery, when the baby comes in contact with the mother's blood in her vagina. If the mother takes antiretroviral medicines during the delivery, and/or if the baby is delivered by caesarean section (a surgical operation to remove the baby from the uterus), the chance that the baby will come in contact with the mother's blood and be infected is much lower.

- If the baby continues taking antiretrovirals for a month after birth, the risk of HIV infection in the baby is even less.

- Finally, the baby at risk of being infected with HIV should be fed only formula, because the mother's breast milk can spread the HIV infection to the baby.

By taking action at any step in this process, the mother can dramatically reduce the risk of passing her infection on to her child. Between 1994 and 2001, the number of cases of HIV transmission from mother to child has been reduced by over 90%.

Keeping the Blood Supply and Transplant Organs HIV-Free

Another mode of HIV transmission, transfusion of blood products or organ transplants, has been virtually eliminated in the United States. This required asking people who knew they had risk factors for HIV infection not to donate blood or organs. Now that methods for diagnosing HIV are readily available, donors are also tested for antibody to HIV. Blood from donors who test positive for HIV or whose results are indeterminate is not used for transfusions.

Because people who are infected with HIV may not have detectable levels of the HIV antibody in their blood for several months, a negative antibody test cannot eliminate the risk that a donor may be infected. For added protection, all donated blood products that are not damaged by heating are treated with heat to kill any HIV. HIV is very sensitive to prolonged heating and cannot survive at temperatures greater than 140°F (60°C). The U.S. Food and Drug Administration requires that all blood products that will not be harmed by heat be heated for 10 to 11 hours at 140° F (60°C).

Manufacturers and blood banks have developed other strategies to remove viruses that may not have been detected by testing the donor, including adding chemicals that kill viruses and then removing these chemicals before transfusion. For a certain clotting factor, called Factor VIII, for use by hemophiliacs, an antibody to Factor VIII is placed in a column and blood is passed through the column. The Factor VIII molecules stick to the antibody and the rest of the blood materials pass through, including any viruses. The Factor VIII molecules are then separated from the antibody and prepared as pure Factor VIII for hemophiliacs. For over 10 years, no proven cases of HIV transmission by blood products have occurred in the United States. In some areas, all blood specimens are also tested with PCR.

ASSISTANCE FOR THOSE INFECTED WITH HIV

Once a person is infected with HIV, it is critical to delay as long as possible the progression to AIDS and death, and to reduce his or her risk of transmitting the infection to others. Among the most important strategies is to ensure that every person who has ever had sex with or had any other exposure to the infected person that may result in HIV infection be tested for HIV. All people who have HIV infection are encouraged to accept evaluation and treatment so they will not progress to severe immune suppression. These treatments, because they reduce the amount of HIV in the blood, may actually decrease how infectious they are.

Many other types of assistance are valuable for reducing the risk of new infections. Assisting people with HIV infection to obtain shelter and food, and providing treatment for substance dependence if it is needed, can greatly reduce their risk of transmitting HIV through exchanging sex for shelter or food, or by sharing injection equipment. Providing people who have HIV infection with condoms and sterile needles also reduces the risk of their spreading HIV infection.

It is difficult to estimate how many new HIV infections worldwide have been prevented by treating STDs, abstinence, monogamy with uninfected partners, condom use, and clean needle programs; however, the number is believed to be at least in the hundreds of thousands and probably millions.

8

The Future of HIV/AIDS

No one can predict what is going to happen with the HIV pandemic, but some educated guesses can be made. HIV is not an easy virus to transmit. As we continue to treat diseases that promote the spread of HIV, HIV transmission may decrease. In addition, practices that decrease the spread of HIV infection, particularly the use of latex condoms, are effective in decreasing the number of new HIV infections. The promotion of abstinence, monogamy with an uninfected partner, and condom use among people who have sex with partners who may be infected has dramatically decreased HIV transmission in some of the hardest hit countries in the world, including Uganda and Thailand.

PROMISING PREVENTION METHODS

Several new strategies are being explored to help prevent HIV infection. These include:

- Microbicides

- Lactobacilli

- Post-exposure treatments with antiretroviral drugs.

Microbicides

Microbicides are products that receptive partners of people who may have HIV infection can use to protect themselves from HIV infection. Sometimes called invisible condoms, these products are

(continued on page 118)

INVISIBLE CONDOMS: HOW VAGINAL MICROBICIDES MIGHT WORK

Since the late 1980s, when male latex condoms where shown to be very effective in preventing sexual spread of HIV infection, a substitute was sought for people who cannot or will not use condoms. The main substitutes have been products (e.g., gels, creams, and suppositories) called microbicides (meaning "killers of microorganisms") that may be placed in the vagina or rectum to protect against infection. Many microbicides are in various stages of testing right now.

Unlike antiretrovirals, microbicides work *before* infection, while HIV is in the vagina or rectum, to either inactivate HIV or prevent HIV from getting a foothold in the vulnerable cells (the ones that have the handles onto which HIV can bind). Most of the microbicides that are in development work to enhance the vagina's natural protector, acidity. Others work as **surfactants**.

Surfactants actually kill HIV in the vagina. Unfortunately, the experience with nonoxynol-9 showed that some products that kill HIV damage the protective lining of the vagina, actually making the lining more vulnerable to HIV. Chorhexidine Gel (ZnG-Gel™) is one surfactant being tested.

Other microbicides that protect vaginal tissues from HIV infection include **adsorption inhibitors**, **entry and fusion inhibitors**, and **replication inhibitors**.

- Adsorption inhibitors make it hard for HIV to get close to vulnerable cells. Examples of this type of microbicide include Carraguard™, made from a seaweed material added to many puddings, milkshakes, and other desserts as carrageenan, and dextrin-2-sulfate.

- **Entry and fusion inhibitors** prevent the attachment and membrane merging, which start infection. These include CCR5 inhibitors and a CD4+ protein. These chemicals tie up HIV that might otherwise bind to real CD4 or CCR5 on cells.

- **Replication inhibitors** are antiretrovirals. They include some that are often used by people who already have HIV. But for microbicide use, they are made into pills or creams that are put into the vagina or rectum. They would block multiplication of HIV that has managed to get into vulnerable cells so they will not produce more HIV that can infect other cells.

(continued from page 116)

gels, creams, or other products that people at risk can put into the vagina or rectum to protect these tissues from infection. While microbicides are not as effective as mechanical barriers such as condoms, they may be a lifesaving alternative for people who cannot or will not use condoms.

Lactobacilli

For women, one of the most innovative concepts in protection is recolonizing the vagina with acid-producing microorganisms called **lactobacilli**, which are normal inhabitants of the healthy vagina (Figure 8.1). Some lactobacilli normally make the vagina very resistant to STDs, particularly HIV. This idea is very exciting because lactobacilli do not have to be used every time a woman has intercourse or even every week. Lactobacilli can be put in a capsule that is placed in the vagina. After the capsule has been in the vagina for a few days, the vagina will be colonized with lactobacilli, which provide protection for a

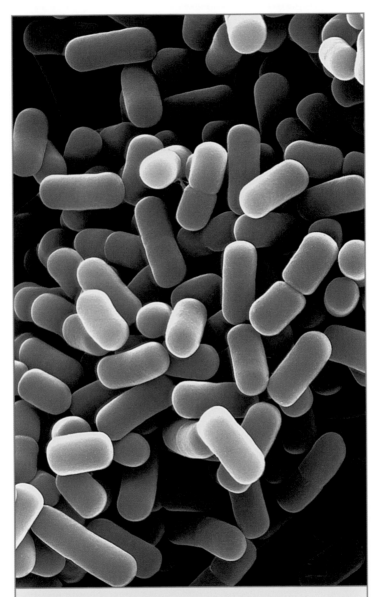

Figure 8.1 Gram-positive rods called lactobacilli (shown here) colonize the vagina, making it inhospitable to HIV and other sexually transmitted microorganisms. Scientists are researching the possibility of using lactobacilli as a preventive measure against certain STDs.

month or more. Because most healthy women already have lactobacilli in their systems, this treatment would not interfere with pregnancy.

POST-EXPOSURE TREATMENTS WITH ANTIRETROVIRAL DRUGS

A very controversial prevention strategy is the use of post-exposure treatments to reduce the risk of HIV infection after exposure. Antiretroviral treatment is administered as soon as a person realizes that he or she may have been exposed to HIV.

THE "GOOD BUG" PEOPLE

Could bacteria help protect women from HIV? That was the question that prompted a now 10-year-old research effort by two microbiologists, Drs. Gerald Chrisope and Sharon Hillier.

The mucous membranes of female genitals have formidable defenses against HIV. But worldwide, these defenses are breached daily, resulting in thousands of new sexual transmissions of HIV each week. If these natural defenses could be fortified, perhaps fewer women would become infected.

One of the main normal defense mechanisms is a bacterium called *Lactobacillus* (literally, "milk bacterium"), which produces acids. Lactobacilli are found normally in the mouth, vagina, and intestinal mucous membranes, all of which are potential entry points for many harmful microorganisms.

About 40% of women have species of lactobacilli that make hydrogen peroxide and acids. These chemicals make the vagina downright dangerous for harmful microorganisms. Women in whom lactobacilli are replaced by other microorganisms, a condition called bacterial vaginosis, are more prone to infection by HIV. If these women could be

This strategy has probably prevented some HIV infections. Post-exposure treatments appeared to decrease the risk of HIV infection in health-care workers who were stuck with needles used to treat people with advanced HIV infection, and possibly even in people who had unprotected sex with a person with HIV. However, for this treatment to work, antiretrovirals must be used less than 72 hours after exposure, and use of antiretrovirals always carries a risk. At least one person has died and one person has suffered permanent side effects due to antiretroviral treatment to prevent HIV infection.

given lactobacillis treatments to restore the natural balance of bacteria, they might be less prone to HIV infection.

In the laboratory, protective chemicals produced by these harmless bacteria destroy HIV and other harmful microorganisms. Dr. Chrisope reasoned that a product made from these bacteria, a probiotic, could help prevent HIV. Dr. Hillier obtained strains of lactobacillus from many healthy women. One strain produced many grams of protective chemicals per day. This strain was rigorously tested and was found to kill harmful microorganisms effectively. Here was a product that would not need to be used every time a woman had sex, or even every week! It would only be placed into the vagina twice a day for three days, and then it would colonize the vagina, and protect it for at least a month.

Initial studies after treatment for bacterial vaginosis yielded mixed results; only 70% of women who took the probiotic were colonized with the beneficial bacteria. Those women were protected against the return of bacterial vaginosis, but the other 30% were not. Dr. Chrisope and Dr. Hillier went "back to the drawing board," trying to find a way around the glitch. They are now working hard on a modified version of the lactobacillus preparation, to see if it is more effective.

EXPLORING THE POSSIBILITY OF AN HIV VACCINE

Researchers are working to develop a vaccine to prevent infection by HIV. Developing an HIV vaccine poses great challenges. The most effective vaccines trigger a significant antibody response. Infection with HIV results in a strong antibody response against HIV's glycoprotein-120. It seems that the antibody response helps control the virus, at least for some years. However, rising levels of HIV eventually overwhelm the antibody response, leading to uncontrolled infection, even in the presence of the antibody. The vaccine must avoid the unknown pitfalls that limit the protective effect of the natural antibody.

Recently, more has been discovered about why the protective effects of neutralizing antibodies eventually wane. Alabama researchers showed that in the early weeks of infection, the neutralizing antibodies work very well. After a while, however, the antibodies, like antiretrovirals, start to encounter resistant mutants. Having killed off viruses that are sensitive to the antibodies allows resistant mutants to reproduce unchecked. These viruses then give rise to billions of viruses that are completely resistant to the antibodies.

HIV can be transmitted as free viral particles, but also within infected cells. For a vaccine to be effective, it must protect against both forms of the virus. Although vaccines are generally considered preventive strategies, HIV vaccine candidates are being tested both as preventive and treatment (therapeutic) products. **Preventive vaccines**, given to people who are not infected, would work by protecting the person from getting infected with HIV. **Therapeutic vaccines**, given to people who are already infected with HIV, would try to improve the way the immune system works even though it is hampered by the infection.

Some vaccines that are being tested work to boost the cell-mediated immune response to HIV. One vaccine candidate uses synthetic components of HIV to incite killer T cells to destroy HIV infected cells. T cells attack these chemicals, which they perceive as being pieces of HIV. Because these chemicals just *look* like HIV, but are not actually HIV, they cannot cause HIV infection.

Frustration on the Way to Developing an HIV Vaccine

Dr. Donald Francis, one of the main CDC investigators of the AIDS epidemic in 1981, also explored the possibility of an HIV vaccine. More than 5,417 HIV-negative volunteers, 5,108 of them homosexual men, received the vaccine in seven injections given for more than three years. Approximately one-third of the participants received a placebo. More than 90% of the participants kept up with their regimens. The FDA had stated that if the vaccine lowered the risk of getting HIV infection by only 30%, it would be good enough to license the product. Many HIV epidemiologists believed that even if it lowered the risk by only 20%, it would be very helpful in places with very high HIV prevalence, particularly if, at the same time, condom use increased.

Unfortunately, almost 58 of each 1,000 people in the trial who received placebo and 57 of each 1,000 who received the vaccine got infected. The difference was, of course, not significant. It will be some time before all the details of the trial findings are analyzed. Some early analyses suggest that in some groups, the effects of the vaccine were much better than in the group overall.

The main problem confronting vaccine researchers is similar to the problem faced by those researchers working on antiretrovirals. There are well-defined viral targets of attack, but many of the targets that produce the biggest surge of antibody or killer T cells change rapidly and become unrecognizable to the immune system.

Because vaccines contain synthetic parts of HIV, they cannot cause HIV infection or AIDS in trial participants.

(continued on page 125)

HOPE FROM A FAMOUS VIRUS HUNTER

One of the scientists who worked on the 1981 investigation of the first AIDS cases was a medical epidemiologist at the CDC named Donald Francis. Dr. Francis, a virologist and physician, worked all over the world investigating epidemics, helping to eradicate smallpox, control cholera and Ebola virus, and develop the hepatitis B vaccine, one of the most successful vaccines in medical history. He was one of the first to suggest that AIDS was an infectious disease and to realize what HIV would do to our country and the world.

His most recent projects include working on an HIV vaccine. HIV needs a surface protein to enter cells. Antibodies to that protein seem to counteract (neutralize) the ability of the virus to enter cells. Dr. Francis reasoned that if the antibody were ready and waiting for HIV, it might stop HIV from being able to cause infection.

As Dr. Francis prepared to test his vaccine, thousands of people who were HIV-negative volunteered for his studies. His idea was to vaccinate people who did not have HIV infection with a protein that looked to the immune system just like one of the proteins on the surface of HIV. This vaccine would be given to people who were at very high risk of getting HIV infection. To determine if the vaccine actually prevented HIV infection, the vaccine was given to some volunteers and a placebo, or inactive vaccine, was given to others.

In this study, twice as many volunteers received the vaccine than the placebo. At the end of the study, the two groups were compared. The hope was that those who received vaccine would have a lower infection rate those who received the placebo.

Overall, very few people in either group became infected. The rate of acquiring HIV infection was much lower than expected. As part of the study, the researchers had encouraged the participants to assume they were taking the placebo. They were warned to make sure that they were using the most effective HIV prevention that they could. Most people carefully used condoms when they had sex. The study findings indicated that the people who received the vaccine were only slightly less likely to become infected than those who received the placebo.

Researchers discovered some interesting patterns when they looked at specific subgroups of participants. For example, 8% of black people who received the placebo became infected. The infection rate for other ethnicities was less than 6%. Less than 2% of black people who received the active vaccine became infected. This means that black people who received the vaccine had a risk of HIV infection that was 78% lower than placebo users, a statistically significant difference. The data from this study are being analyzed, but it is doubtful that this vaccine will receive further testing. Another study of this vaccine in Thailand failed to show a protective effect. Meanwhile, other vaccines are also being tested.

(continued from page 123)

A company called Epimmune Inc. recently announced that it started human trials for preliminary safety of a preventive HIV vaccine, EP HIV-1090, in the United States and Africa. This trial plans to enroll 42 volunteers at sites in New England and Botswana. Epimmune is also testing the vaccine to treat people with HIV in human trials for preliminary and expanded safety that began in the United States in September 2002.

9

Conclusion

As we conclude this book, there is much reason for disappointment. It is not just that the first vaccine trial was unsuccessful. It is not just that we are years from having a truly effective microbicide on the market. It is not just that the number of AIDS cases has started to climb again. What is really troubling is that for many people, HIV has become a nonissue, not as important as whatever has caught the national attention at present. The promotion of preventive strategies that work very well has become the subject of political tugs of war. In some countries, unfounded fears that condoms promote sexual risk drive policy to make them harder for at-risk people to acquire. In other countries, such as South Africa, use of antiretrovirals to prevent mother-to-child trans-mission continues to be restricted.

However, there is also reason for hope. Dr. Ward Cates said in 1985 that any person with any sense of history can tell that AIDS has the potential to be the worst thing to happen to humankind. Yet, any person with any sense of the past can also tell that some good things have come out of the HIV epidemic. For many people who were not alive in 1980, this idea may come as a shock. But there was a time when people did not think of the possibility that an infectious disease could cause them serious harm. That view has changed. There was a time when many people in developed countries did not think that anything much that happened in developing countries was a problem for them. That now has also changed.

We must admit that, although this is truly the most catastrophic health crisis in human memory, HIV/AIDS has changed public health for the better. It has forced health professionals to reexamine many dogmas.

(continued on page 128)

Since 1983, a major force in HIV prevention has been a public health physician named Dr. Ron Valdiserri. Ron and his twin brother, Edwin, like most twins, seemed very similar in some ways. They were both physicians, with a rare blend of academic excellence and human warmth. In other ways, they were very different.

Their work fused the ideals of compassion in patient care and rigor in research. Edwin became a psychiatrist and Ron became a pathologist, studying how infections cause disease. Later, Ron entered public health to attempt to study how access to health care and social factors turn infections that are difficult to transmit into epidemics. In the 1980s, both brothers contributed important research about HIV prevention. Some of their work is included in the bibliography of this book.

Dr. Ron Valdiserri was among the first public health scientists to understand the importance of ensuring that prevention scientists understood why people pursued some behaviors and held certain attitudes. He examined how some of these attitudes come from having been treated unfairly in the past. He discovered that there are valid reasons for even some irrational fears and mistrust that have to be addressed.

Dr. Ron Valdiserri went to work at CDC in 1989. Since 1994, he has been deputy director of the National Center for HIV, STDs, and Tuberculosis Prevention at CDC. His mission continues to be, first and foremost, the prevention of HIV. He led the effort of designing the CDC HIV Prevention Strategic Plan through 2005, and oversees its implementation.

Dr. Edwin Valdiserri examined how the fear of getting AIDS could sometimes make people depressed and irrational. It made some believe that AIDS could never happen to them, a condition known as denial. It made others do things that increased their risk of getting HIV, since they believed getting

BUILDING THE FUTURE *(continued)*

the disease was inevitable. He saw the need to take a fresh and compassionate look at the mental health needs of people in prison.

In 1992, Dr. Edwin Valdiserri died of AIDS, leaving a void in the lives of all of us who loved him. But he remains a powerful inspiration through his contributions and the tireless work of his brother.

(continued from page 126)

It has incorporated activism, compassion, and humanity into science that was sorely needed. Whether medical professionals have always welcomed it or not, community members have demanded, and rightfully expect, to have real input in how research is conducted. Patients have an increasing say in how they will be treated. There is increasing appreciation of how tightly the destinies of people worldwide are connected.

The response of the health-care community to infectious diseases that have emerged since HIV first came on the scene is a testimonial to how much medical thinking has changed since the 1980s. From hantavirus to severe acute respiratory syndrome (SARS), the response of the health-care community has been rapid. No time was wasted considering whether enough people had died to make these "serious" health problems. Even problems that affect very poor or marginalized people in other countries are considered serious. HIV has convinced us that the same problems affect people all over the world.

Appendix

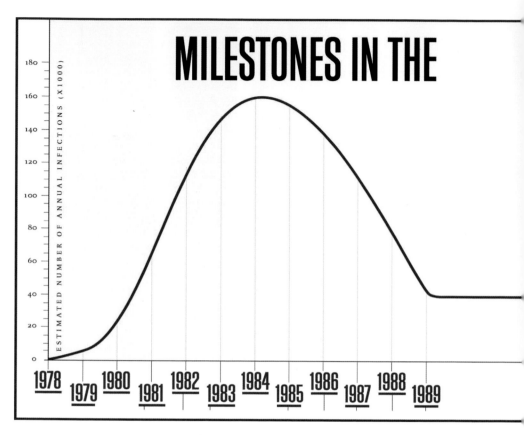

MILESTONES IN THE

| 1978 | 1979 | 1980 | 1981 | 1982 | 1983 | 1984 | 1985 | 1986 | 1987 | 1988 | 1989 |

1981
June 5 First reported cases of *Pneumocystis carinii* pneumonia among men who have sex with men in Los Angeles.

1981–1983 *June 5, 1981–January 7, 1983* All major routes of HIV transmission identified and reported in *MMWR*.

1983
CDC National AIDS Hotline established.

March 4 First prevention recommendations issued by CDC, FDA, and NIH on how to prevent sexual, drug-related, and occupational transmission.

May Human T cell leukemia virus (HTLV) identified in patients with AIDS.

1985
State and local health departments nationwide funded to implement HIV prevention programs.

U.S. HIV EPIDEMIC

CENTERS FOR DISEASE
CONTROL AND PREVENTION

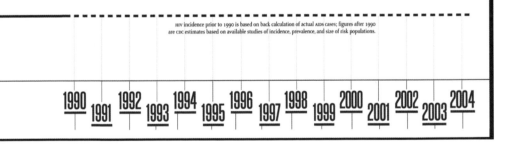

HIV incidence prior to 1990 is based on back calculation of actual AIDS cases; figures after 1990 are CDC estimates based on available studies of incidence, prevalence, and size of risk populations.

1990 1991 1992 1993 1994 1995 1996 1997 1998 1999 2000 2001 2002 2003 2004

January 11 First guidelines for blood screening issued.

March FDA licenses ELISA.

April 15–17 First International Conference on AIDS held.

1986

October 3 Possible transmission from dentist to patient reported.

December 12 HTLV-III is now termed HIV.

1987

America Responds to AIDS, a public information campaign, launched.

Comprehensive school-based education funded.

CDC National AIDS Clearinghouse established.

August 14 First Counseling and Testing Guidelines issued.

Appendix

1988 CDC collaboration with National and Regional Minority Organizations and the faith-based community begins.

May 26 "Understanding AIDS" mailed to all U.S. households.

June 24 Universal Precautions established for health-care workers.

CDC significantly expands state and local prevention funding.

1989 Community-based organizations funded to reach underserved African-American communities.

August 18 First 100,000 cases of AIDS reported.

1990 Congress passes the Americans with Disabilities Act, providing legal protection for people with AIDS and other disabilities.

Ryan White Care Act expands access to treatment.

1992 *December 1* Business Responds to AIDS program launched.

1993 Community planning process instituted to better target local prevention efforts.

August 6 Discordant couples studies show condoms are 98% effective against HIV.

1994 *April 29* Following identification of first preventive regimen, perinatal HIV prevention guidelines issued.

1995 500,000 cases of AIDS reported.

December FDA approves the first protease inhibitor.

1996 Short-course regimen identified for reducing perinatal HIV transmission in the developing world.

1997 *February 28* First decline in AIDS deaths reported.

1998 Congressional Black Caucus provides additional funding for minority prevention programs.

1999   *July* Leadership and Investment in Fighting an Epidemic (LIFE) Initiative introduced to address global AIDS pandemic.

Number of AIDS cases acquired through perinatal transmission declines to 144 annual cases, an all-time low.

2000   *October* Global AIDS Program created to coordinate CDC's international HIV/AIDS programs.

2001   CDC announces new HIV Prevention Strategic Plan to cut annual HIV infections in the United States by half within five years.

For the first time in years, the number of AIDS and syphilis cases rises.

2002   At the International AIDS Conference in Barcelona, Spain, Brazil becomes the first developing country to show a decline in AIDS mortality after offering antiretroviral drugs to all those who need them.

2003   First fusion inhibitor antiretroviral approved by FDA.

2004   Researchers reported in the 11th Conference on Retroviruses and Opportunistic Infections on new classes of antiretroviral drugs that are showing promise in early trials, including a drug that blocks chemokine co-receptor 5 used by HIV to bind to a CD4+ T cell. Another new class includes drugs that block entry of the virus into the cell by preventing the envelope glycoprotein 120 from binding to the cell's CD4 receptors and a third that blocks integration of the HIV "provirus" (DNA based on HIV RNA) into the host cell's DNA.

Glossary

Abstinence—Not engaging in an activity. For example, sexual abstinence involves not engaging in any sexual activities.

Acquired immunodeficiency syndrome (AIDS)—A combination of symptoms, signs, and/or laboratory findings that indicate severe problems with the human body's normal defenses against infections and cancers, normally controlled by the part of the immune system that depends on "helper" thymus (T) lymphocytes. First recognized in 1981, AIDS is caused by infection with the human immunodeficiency virus (HIV).

Activation—Stimulation of a cell of the immune system by contact with an "invading" microorganism, which results in the making of proteins such as antibodies or cytokines to destroy the invader. Activation also results in the cell's dividing to make daughter cells that can fight off the invaders, and other cells that "remember" the invader, should it ever be met again.

Acute—Having a rapid onset and course.

AIDS—Acronym for acquired immunodeficiency syndrome.

AIDS dementia—A condition due to direct damage of brain cells by HIV, which results in losing the ability to remember, followed by loss of ability to speak, walk, and perform other normal functions.

Analogue—A molecule made in the laboratory that is very similar to a naturally occurring molecule.

Anamnestic—The immune system's secondary, very powerful response, after it recognizes a second or later encounter with an antigen.

Antibody—An infection-fighting protein molecule in blood or body fluids that is produced by cells and recognizes a foreign protein (antigen) to help destroy it. Antibodies, known also as immunoglobulins, are manufactured by B lymphocytes (cells in the lymph system) in response to antigens. Each antibody binds only to the antigen that prompted its production. For many diseases, such as chicken pox, measles, and tetanus, antibody shows that the patient is immune and will not be reinfected, or become sick, with the organism. The antibody to HIV appears to lose its protective effect after several years.

Antibody-mediated immunity—The type of immunity that fights invading organisms in body fluids (formerly called "humors" in Latin) with antibodies found in blood plasma and lymph. Also called humoral immunity.

Antibody test—Test that detects antibody produced in reaction to an antigen, such as human immunodeficiency virus (HIV). A test for antibodies to HIV is positive when the infected person's immune system has responded to viral protein or (in the case of infants) if the mother's antibody has crossed the placenta.

Antigen—A substance recognized as foreign by the immune system, which triggers an immune response.

Antiretrovirals—Drugs that block certain viral activities that HIV requires in order to reproduce. In combinations of three or more, these drugs have been shown to lower the amount of virus in the blood (viral load) of an infected person. They cannot completely get rid of the virus or cure HIV infection. However, antiretrovirals increase the number of helper T cells, lengthen the amount of time the patient can live without symptoms, and prevent life-threatening infections with microorganisms that take advantage of a weakened immune system.

B cells (B lymphocytes)—A type of lymphocyte (lymph cell) that develops in the bone marrow without going through the thymus. As a plasma cell, it can later produce antibodies. These cells are found in the bone marrow and spleen. They are part of the "humoral" arm (antibody-mediated immunity) of the immune system (versus the cell-mediated branch).

Blood bank—A facility that collects, processes, stores, and distributes blood to be used in medical treatments. Blood donors give one pint of blood that is checked for antibodies to certain diseases, typed, processed, and given to hospitals and clinics for transfusion into patients of the same or compatible blood type who need blood.

Blood products—Substances derived from whole blood donated to blood banks. Blood products include: red blood cells, granulocytes, platelets, albumin, immune globulin (antibodies), plasma, and clotting factor concentrates.

Glossary

Blood transfusion—Putting whole blood or blood components directly into the bloodstream. Among the blood products that can be transfused are red blood cells, plasma, platelets, and granulocytes, as well as a plasma protein rich in clotting factors.

Caesarean section (C-section)—A procedure in which a baby is delivered through a surgical opening in the mother's lower abdomen and womb (uterus). One in five babies in the United States is delivered by C-section. Babies of mothers with HIV infection are sometimes delivered by C-section to decrease exposure to the mother's blood, and therefore HIV, in the birth process.

Capsid—The protein coat of a virus.

CDC—Centers for Disease Control and Prevention. Lead agency of the Department of Health and Human Services of the federal government of the United States for protecting the health and safety of people at home and abroad. The CDC originated in 1946 to fight malaria and then developed strategies to fight other diseases.

CD4, CD8—See **Cluster designation markers.**

Cell-mediated immunity—Type of immunity that defends against viruses and other microorganisms inside host cells, and against cancers. It involves highly specialized cells that circulate in the blood and lymph system tissue.

Cervix—Mouth of the womb.

Chemokine—A chemical messenger released by T cells that attracts immune cells to sites of infection. Several chemokines interfere with HIV replication by "parking" on the same receptors (handles) on T cells that HIV needs to begin attaching to a cell.

Chemokine co-receptors (CCR)—Receptors (handles), or places for chemokines to "park" on some white blood cells, especially T cells. Chemokines are immune system chemicals. HIV needs to bind to these CCRs to start the process of infecting human cells.

Chronic—Infections or other diseases that are long-lasting, taking months or years to run their course (as opposed to "acute" diseases).

Cluster designation (CD) markers—Any of a number of cell surface markers expressed by white blood cells and used to tell the "story" of the cell. These markers can be recognized by certain antibodies and are named with the initials CD and a number. CD markers show which state of development the cell is in and its work in the immune system. For example, cells that have CD4 in their membranes (CD4+ T cells) are helper T cells.

Colonization—The process by which bacteria or other microorganisms take up residence in mucous membranes or skin but do not cause illness or even infection.

Condom—A rubber or plastic sheath that acts as a barrier to lower the risk of spreading disease-causing microorganisms through sex from an infected sex partner to an uninfected partner, and to lower the risk of the female partner becoming pregnant. Condoms for males consist of a sheath made of latex worn on the penis during sexual intercourse. Condoms for females consist of a sheath made of plastic with two rings, one blind end that covers the cervix (mouth of the womb) and one that stays outside of the vagina.

Cytokines—Chemicals released by T cells in response to contact with antigens that trigger effective responses to destroy invading organisms.

Cytotoxic (cell-killer) T cells—Cells of the cell-mediated (thymus-dependent) immune system that recognize and directly eliminate virus-infected cells. They are also referred to as cell killers.

Deoxyribonucleic acid (DNA)—Acids found in the nucleus of the cell that are the basis of heredity. They are in the shape of a double spiral (also called a double helix), resembling a rotated step-ladder. The two spirals are held together by cross-links ("steps") of chemicals called purines and pyrimidines. Purines (adenine and guanine) link to pyrimidines (thymine and cytosine). The order in which these chemicals are arranged in DNA controls how amino acids are arranged into proteins.

Disability—The inability of a person to do something because of a physical or mental problem.

Glossary

Douches—Preparations of chemicals put into the vagina for "cleaning" the body. The use of vaginal douches can affect the body's natural bacterial flora, making the woman more likely to get infections.

Enzyme—A complex protein used by organisms to catalyze (speed up) a chemical reaction. Usually, the name of the enzyme is the name of the reaction that it speeds up, with the suffix "-ase." For example, reverse transcriptase is the enzyme that catalyzes reverse transcription of RNA to DNA.

Enzyme-linked immunosorbent assay (ELISA)—A test (or "assay") for antibody to an organism that works by linking an enzyme to an antibody produced in the laboratory. This antigen to which this laboratory-produced antibody binds is the antibody that the test detects. When the laboratory-produced antibody finds and binds to the antibody in a sample, the enzyme speeds up a color reaction that signals that the sample is "positive" for the test antibody.

Epidemic—The occurrence of more than the expected number of cases of a disease, disease outcome, or other health event in a population. Occurrence of even one case of a disease that is normally not expected, has never been seen before, an occurrance of the disease in people in whom it is not usually seen, or with a death rate that is higher than expected can constitute an epidemic.

Epidemiology—A branch of medical science that deals with the occurrence, spread, and control of disease in a population.

Food and Drug Administration (FDA)—An agency of the federal government of the United States that informs physicians and the public about health risks related to food or medicines. FDA's mission controls research to make sure that medicines are tested for safety and effectiveness in a thorough and timely manner before they are approved for use and continues to monitor them after they are in use.

Fusion—The process by which HIV's viral envelope blends with the cell membrane to allow HIV to insert its nucleic acid inside the cell that it is invading.

Fusion inhibitors—A class of antiretroviral drugs that work by preventing HIV from entering cells in the first place (in contrast to other classes of antiretrovirals, which block HIV activities once it is already inside the cell). Fusion inhibitors are complex and difficult to produce and administer, but they often work when other drugs to combat HIV/AIDS fail.

Gay—See **Homosexual**.

Gene—The hereditary determinant of a characteristic of an individual that is passed through nucleic acid from parent to offspring; sections of several nucleotide "steps" in DNA controlling the passing of a trait from parents to offspring.

Genetic material—Nucleic acids in the nucleus that determine characteristics inherited from parents to offsprings; determined by the genes.

Glycoprotein—A chemical that contains both a protein and a sugar. The HIV coat includes glycoprotein molecules. Glycoproteins can serve as "antigens" (proteins recognized as foreign by the immune system, which trigger very specific responses).

Granulocytes—White blood cells that have granules (little grains) containing chemicals that kill microorganisms.

HAART—See **Highly active antiretroviral therapy**.

Harm reduction—Method of HIV/AIDS prevention that both tries to reduce the harmful effects of high-risk behavior and to reduce the behaviors themselves.

Helper T cell—The principal cell of the cell-mediated immune system. A type of lymphocyte (lymph cell) that has to mature in the thymus and has cluster designation (CD) marker 4 (CD4+). It is required by some B cells to make antibodies and helps other T cells respond to antigens. It protects against many disease-causing microorganisms and cancers.

Hemophilia—A genetic disease in which the blood does not clot because it does not have enough clotting factors, chemicals that quickly stop bleeding. The disease almost exclusively affects males. The disease causes a large amount of bleeding even after small bumps and injuries and, thus, hemophilia can lead to serious internal bleeding, crippling diseases, and death.

Hepatitis G virus—A harmless virus seen more frequently in people who do not get HIV infection than in infected people, and in people with very slow progression from HIV infection to AIDS. Hepatitis G is sometimes found in people infected with HIV or with hepatitis C. Hepatitis G causes no disease and may somehow improve survival in HIV.

Heterosexual—A person who is sexually attracted to members of the opposite sex.

Highly active antiretroviral therapy—Also known as HAART, an antiretroviral regimen containing a combination of at least three antiretroviral medicines that can lower the amount of HIV in the blood to less than the level that the best tests can detect and raise the number of T cells to over 200 in patients with HIV infection.

Highly exposed, persistently seronegative (uninfected)—Also known as HEPS, people who are at high risk for infection with HIV, but who, over a long period of time, do not get infected. They engage in high-risk sexual behaviors with infected persons but remain uninfected.

Homosexual—A person who is sexually attracted to members of his or her own sex. Homosexual men are also called "gays." Homosexual women are also called "lesbians."

Human immunodeficiency virus (HIV)—Any of the various mutations of the HIV virus, especially HIV-1, that infect and destroy helper T cells of the immune system. Also called the AIDS virus. HIV-1 is the subtype of HIV that causes most cases of AIDS. One of a class of retroviruses, which have genes composed of ribonucleic acid (RNA) molecules and use an enzyme called reverse transcriptase to convert their RNA into DNA, which is then incorporated into the host cell's DNA.

Human papillomavirus—A family of viruses that includes subtypes that cause skin and genital warts, and some cancers. Only a small proportion of persons with normal immune systems who get infected with these viruses develop cancers or even warts. However, many people whose immune systems are weakened by HIV and are infected with human papillomavirus will get warts or cancers from it.

Humoral immunity—See **Antibody-mediated immunity**.

Immune response—Response of the immune system to an antigen.

Immunodeficiency—A condition in which the immune system is prevented from protecting the host from antigens.

Immunosuppression—A curbing of the ability of the immune system to protect the host from antigens.

Infection—A process in which a microorganism enters a host and uses some of the host cell's function for its own survival and multiplication.

Infectious disease—A disease or organ malfunction caused by infection with a microorganism.

Inflammation—From the Latin for "setting on fire." A complex reaction of body and tissue cells to infection or injury, to contain invading microorganisms by increasing blood flow to the area, bringing cells to the area that can release chemicals, raising the temperature, and otherwise defending the host against invading microorganisms.

Infrastructure of public health—The foundation or basic framework for the monitoring and protection of the health of people within a country. This includes staff, buildings, equipment, and supplies required to deliver services.

Injection drug use—Using a needle to place a drug in the body. Tiny amounts of blood usually stay in the needle or syringe after a person uses it for injection drug use. If that person has HIV or another blood-borne infection, people who use the needle or syringe after the infected person can get infected as well.

Kaposi's sarcoma—A type of cancer caused by abnormal growth of blood vessels that swell into purplish or brown lesions. This cancer is caused by human herpes virus 8 (HHV-8). Humans have always had this virus, which can be sexually transmitted. In people with normal immune systems, it poses little risk. However, when the immune system is weakened by HIV, the HHV-8 virus causes a deadly cancer. The severe form of Kaposi's sarcoma is one of the opportunistic infections that can occur in a person infected by HIV, causing purplish growths on the skin, lymph nodes, stomach, intestines, lungs, liver, and spleen.

Lactobacilli—Acid-producing microorganisms that normally live in a healthy vagina.

Latent—Potentially existing, but not active or visible. HIV infection at the cellular level is never really latent. However, in terms of signs and symptoms ("clinically"), HIV infection when acquired during adulthood usually goes through a latent period that may last up to 10 years.

Lentivirinae—Latin for "slow-acting viruses." Subfamily of retroviruses that cause chronic sexually transmitted or blood-borne infectious diseases with long periods of time when the infected person has no symptoms.

Lymph—A colorless fluid derived from blood, which circulates in the lymphatic system, similar to the circulatory system. Lymph is collected by drainage from the tissues throughout the body, flows in the lymph vessels through the lymph nodes, and then is added to the blood in the veins. Lymph carries some white blood cells (mostly lymphocytes).

Lymph nodes—Tiny oval organs varying in diameter from 0.1 to 2.5 centimeters which act as barriers to infection by filtering out harmful microorganisms that enter the body through blood, cuts in the skin, and mucous membranes. More than 100 are normally found in the body, mainly in the neck, groin, armpits, and along the lymph vessels. Within the lymph nodes, white blood cells can destroy these microorganisms and their products.

Lymphocytes—From the Latin for "lymph cell." White blood cells present in lymph responsible for the immune response, which protects the human body from harmful microorganisms and cancers.

Macrophage—An amoeba-like cell that moves through tissues, engulfing bacteria, viruses, and dead cells. Macrophages stimulate other immune system cells by presenting them with small pieces of the invaders to prompt an immune response.

Memory cells—Long-lived B or T lymphocytes that are "saved" during the first encounter with an antigen for subsequent encounters with the same antigen. B cells that, after a first encounter with an antigen and activation, do not differentiate into plasma cells. Instead, they undergo DNA rearrangements, so that the next time they encounter the antigen, they quickly make large amounts of specialized IgG, IgA, or IgE antibody. T cells that do not get involved in the attack on an antigen during the first encounter, instead acting as the filing system to record that a particular antigen has been previously met. They are the cell pool for future multiplication into many activated cells to mount an effective response should a reencounter occur.

Men who have sex with men—Men who have physical sexual activities (versus attraction or orientation) with other men, regardless of reason. Although many of these men are homosexual, some are, or think of themselves as, bisexual or heterosexual.

Microorganisms—Living beings that cannot be seen with the naked eye.

Microbicides—Gels, creams, or other products put into the vagina or rectum to protect the tissues from infection.

Molecular weights—The weight of a molecule in atomic mass units calculated by adding the atomic weights of each element in the compound.

Monogamy—Having only one sexual partner.

***Morbidity and Mortality Weekly Report* (*MMWR*)**—A newsletter prepared weekly by the Centers for Disease Control and Prevention (CDC). The information in the *MMWR* includes up-to-date reports of trends based on weekly reports to the CDC by state health departments.

Glossary

Mucous membranes—The lubricated inner lining of the mouth, nasal passages, vagina, intestines, and urethra (tube that drains the bladder of urine); any membrane or lining that contains mucus-secreting glands.

Mucus—A sticky, slippery secretion that is usually rich in mucins or proteins; it is produced by the mucous membranes that it moistens, lubricates, and protects.

Mutant—Individual that results from a gene or chromosome spontaneously changing its structure as it reproduces (mutation).

Mutation—A spontaneous change in a gene's structure or number, resulting in some change in the function or structure of the substance for which the gene codes.

Mycobacterium tuberculosis—The bacterium that causes tuberculosis (TB), an infectious, chronic disease that commonly affects the lungs, although it may occur in almost any part of the body. The most common mode of transmission of tuberculosis is inhalation of air with dried, suspended bacteria released by people with tuberculosis of the lung when they cough, sneeze, or speak.

Naïve cells—Lymphocytes that have never encountered the type of antigen to which, genetically, they are able to respond.

Natural killer (NK) cells—Lymphocytes that do not require any prior encounter with an antigen to be able to destroy invading microorganisms.

Natural selection—A process by which certain organisms are "chosen" to survive because they have developed the ability to withstand the effect of a substance(s) that kills other members of its species, usually due to a mutation. When an antiretroviral drug is taken by a patient with HIV infection, it kills all HIV that cannot withstand (or "resist") the effects of the medicine. Any resistant HIV can then multiply without competition. The antiretroviral thus "selects" the resistant mutants.

Non-nucleoside reverse transcriptase inhibitors (NNRTIs)—Class of HIV medicines that inhibit (block) the action of the viral enzyme reverse transcriptase. Drugs in this class include Efavirenz and Nevirapine, and only need to be taken once a day.

Nucleic acids (NA)—A molecule composed of nucleotides that are joined by bonds between the phosphate group of one nucleotide and the sugar of the next nucleotide. The principal nucleic acids are ribonucleic and deoxyribonucleic acids (RNA and DNA).

Nucleoside reverse transcriptase inhibitors (NRTIs)—Class of HIV medicines that inhibit (block) the action of the viral enzyme reverse transcriptase, by tricking it into using the drug as one of the nucleosides (adenine, thymidine, cytosine, or guanine). Drugs in this class include Zidovudine (azidothymidine, an analogue for thymidine), and ddC (an analogue for cytosine).

Nucleus—A structure inside a cell surrounded by a membrane that contains the cell's genetic material.

Opportunistic infection—An infection that would not cause disease if the individual did not have immunodeficiency. An opportunistic infection takes advantage of the fact that the body's normal defenses are down, giving it an opportunity to cause disease. One example that is often seen in AIDS patients is *Pneumocystis carinii* pneumonia.

Pandemic—A disease prevalent throughout an entire country, continent, or the whole world. In the 21st century, HIV/AIDS is pandemic.

Placebo—An inactive substance, such as a sugar pill, used in drug studies to help determine if the drug actually has a real effect.

Placebo-controlled study—A study that controls for "placebo effect" by assigning some study participants the drug or treatment being tested, and others a placebo that is similar in appearance to the drug. The participants do not know whether they are taking the placebo or the drug being tested. The placebo effect is the tendency to feel better when taking even an inactive substance. Results for the two groups must differ significantly to determine that the drug or treatment actually works.

***Pneumocystis carinii* pneumonia**—Pneumonia due to infection of the lungs by *Pneumocystis carinii*, a fungus. In people with normal immune systems, *P. carinii* is often found growing at low levels harmlessly in the lungs. However, it grows rapidly in people with severe cell-mediated immunodeficiency. It is the most frequent severe AIDS-related opportunistic infection, and a frequent cause of death.

Polymorphonuclear leukocyte—A white blood cell that typically defends against infection by phagocytosis or antibody production.

Precursor protein—One of nine HIV proteins that are large and inactive when first made, and become active when cut down into smaller proteins by HIV protease enzymes.

Prenatal care—Care of a pregnant woman before delivery of the child to prevent complications of pregnancy and promote a healthy outcome for both mother and child.

Preventive vaccines—Vaccines (immunizations) that prevent an infectious disease by presenting to the immune system a harmless antigen that is very similar to a disease-causing microorganism or its products, so that if the person is then exposed to the real microorganism, a powerful anamnestic response will prevent infection.

Primary response—The first response to an antigen appearing within 7 to 10 days after infection. Induced by naïve lymphocytes to an antigen that the immune system has never before encountered. The production of antibody (mostly immunoglobulin M [IgM]), after the first encounter between an antigen and a B lymphocyte, when some B lymphocytes activated by contact with the antigen become plasma cells, dedicated to making IgM antibody. Similarly, the response to activation of naïve T lymphocytes by antigen-presenting cells during a first encounter with an antigen, when they multiply in numbers and go to sites to produce inflammation and control the invasion.

Protease—An enzyme that breaks down proteins into their short strands of amino acids (peptides). HIV's protease enzyme breaks apart long strands of inactive viral protein into the separate active proteins making up the viral core.

Protease inhibitors (PIs)—An antiviral drug that acts to interrupt the budding of a new HIV cell. If the larger HIV proteins are not broken apart, they cannot assemble themselves into new HIV particles.

Provirus—Viral DNA that inserts into a host cell's DNA.

Reactivated, reactivation—A term often used in regard to tuberculosis. After initial (primary) infection with *Mycobacterium tuberculosis*, T cells will control the organism, making the infection latent (inactive). In up to 10% of normal adults, and virtually all young infants and persons with HIV infection, the *M. tuberculosis* organisms overwhelm the immune response and multiply rapidly if untreated with antituberculosis medicines. The disease caused by this resurgence is called "reactivation."

Reject—A process by which the T cells of the body, after recognizing that an organ or tissue is foreign (not "self," as in a transplant), will go to the foreign tissue and destroy it.

Replication—Making more cells by dividing, while preserving all of the qualities of the parent cells, so that the daughter cells are "copies" of the parent cells.

Resistance—The ability of a microorganism to withstand the effects of a drug that is deadly to most members of its species.

Retroviral syndrome—An illness that occurs in about a third of people within 6 weeks after they are first infected with HIV. HIV infection at this point is easily mistaken for another viral infection such as flu. Symptoms, including sore throat, headache, muscle aches, joint pains, enlarged lymph nodes, rash, nausea, vomiting, or diarrhea, usually disappear on their own after 2 to 3 weeks. Also known as seroconversion syndrome.

Retrovirus—An RNA virus that reproduces by changing its RNA into DNA using an enzyme called reverse transcriptase, and then inserting the DNA into the host cell's chromosome.

Reverse transcriptase—An enzyme made by some RNA viruses that uses RNA as a template (pattern) to make DNA that can be placed into the host cell's DNA. This enzyme of HIV and other retroviruses converts the single-stranded viral RNA into DNA, the form in which the cell carries its genes.

Reverse transcriptase inhibitors (RTIs)—A class of antiviral drugs that block the action of reverse transcriptase in the infected cell.

Glossary

Ribonucleic acid (RNA)—A nucleic acid containing ribose as the sugar within the nucleotides. The genetic storage material of some viruses. Used by animal and plant cells to translate the genetic instructions in the nuclear DNA into specific instructions for making all the proteins the organism needs.

Risk factors—Characteristics found more commonly among people with a condition under study ("cases") than in those who are similar to cases, but do not have the condition under study ("controls").

Risk groups—Groups whose members include those with risk factors for a specific condition.

Routes of transmission—The mode of spread for a microorganism. For HIV, the common routes of transmission include sexual, mother-to-child, and through blood.

"Safer" sex—Sexual activities that, compared to activities very likely to promote HIV transmission, have lower risk, or are "safer." Safer sexual activities include avoiding sexual activities where persons come into contact with the other partner's potentially infectious body fluids, such as blood or genital fluids.

Secondary response—The more rapid, stronger, and longer-lasting response when the immune system encounters an antigen a second or later time.

Seroconversion syndrome—See **Retroviral syndrome**.

Serum—The clear, watery part of the blood plasma that remains after clots have formed and been removed. Contains antibodies.

Sexual transmission—Spread of a microorganism through sexual acts.

Sexually transmitted diseases (STDs)—Diseases or infections, also called venereal diseases (VDs) or sexually transmitted infections (STIs), caused by organisms that are usually spread from person to person during sex, including syphilis, gonorrhea, chlamydia, and many others.

Simian immunodeficiency virus—A retrovirus that can cause immunodeficiency whose host species is a type of ape or monkey.

Spermicides—Chemicals in birth control creams and jellies, and sometimes added to vaginal sponges or condoms, that kill sperm cells.

Strain—A genetic "version" of an organism. Many viruses, including HIV, exist in population as one of many versions of the species or subspecies. Because HIV mutates so frequently and multiplies so rapidly, many different strains quickly emerge.

Suppressor T cell—A type of T cell that causes B cells as well as other cells to ignore antigens. T lymphocytes responsible for turning the immune response off after an infection is cleared. They are CD8+ lymphocytes (lymphocytes with surface cluster designation [CD]8).

Surfactants—Products that kill HIV after it enters the vagina.

Synergistic—When things that interact with each other in such a way that the total effect being greater than the sum of the individual effects. Some drugs are synergistic; that is, they work together to create an effect that neither drug would have alone. Some diseases are synergistic, too, having much more impact together than the sum of their individual effects.

Syphilis—A chronic infectious disease caused by a bacterium, *Treponema pallidum*, usually transmitted by sexual contact or from mother to infant during pregnancy. If left untreated, syphilis produces genital ulcers and body rashes, and severe late-stage lesions over many years, and also promotes HIV transmission.

T cell (T lymphocyte)—A white blood cell that arises from the lymph-cell stem cells that has to pass through the thymus to mature completely (thymus cell). In the thymus, it loses one CD-marker from its surface, either CD-8 or CD-4, to become a CD4+ ("helper") or CD8+ ("suppressor") T cell.

Glossary

Therapeutic vaccines—A type of immunization given to persons who already have an infection, to try to treat the infection by strengthening the immune response against the microorganism. The vaccine contains chemicals that cause the antigen to trigger a stronger response, which will then be directed at the organism causing the infection.

Thymus—A gland made mostly of lymphoid tissue that helps in the development of the body's immune system. The thymus is located in the upper chest or at the base of the neck and tends to shrink in adulthood. T lymphocytes go through a maturation process in the thymus from which only about 5% emerge.

Toxin—A poisonous substance sometimes made by harmful micro-organisms that can cause disease and trigger antibody formation when encountered by an organism's immune system.

Transcription—In cell biology, the use of a nucleic acid pattern by the cell to construct a matching nucleic acid.

Transfusion—Putting whole blood or blood components directly into the bloodstream of a patient to treat various conditions, such as shock from blood loss or severe anemia. Blood components include packed red blood cells, plasma, platelets, granulocytes, and plasma protein rich in clotting factors to prevent bleeding in people with hemophilia.

Transplants—Placing a healthy organ from a living donor or someone who has died to replace a damaged organ in another person. Common transplants include kidney, liver, lungs, heart, and corneas.

Tuberculosis (TB)—A chronic infectious disease of humans caused by the bacterium *Mycobacterium tuberculosis*. It has a primary stage, usually a mild pneumonia, to which the body responds with cell-mediated immune response, driving the organisms into lymph nodes, where they remains latent (inactive). Reactivation into pulmonary tuberculosis, or tuberculosis in other organs, occurs in about 10% of normal people over the following years, and in close to 100% of people with HIV.

Tubo-ovarian abscesses—Pus-filled lesions caused by infection, usually due to gonorrhea or, less often, by *Chlamydia trachomatis*, which has risen from the mouth of the womb (cervix) into the womb, fallopian tubes, and ovaries.

Upregulate—Increase the activity of HIV or suseptibility of cells to becoming infected, usually by providing more chemokine co-receptors for binding to cells.

Virion—The complete viral particle, found outside of a cell and capable of surviving in crystalline form and infecting another living cell. It is made up of the nucleid core (genetic material) and the capsid (protein shell that protects the nucleic acid).

Virus—The causative agents of multiple infectious diseases. Any of a large group of infective agents that contain a protein coat surrounding a core of genetic material. Viruses cannot grow and multiply on their own. They must be within living cells to multiply. They are only visible with electron microscopes and are smaller than bacteria.

Zidovudine—First drug approved for treatment of HIV infection. FDA approval was granted in 1987 for use with advanced HIV disease in adults and in 1990 for pediatric use. Zidovudine used in combination with other drugs delays the complications of HIV infection by many months or years, and alone can decrease the risk of mother-to-child transmission.

Bibliography

Anderson, Jean, ed. *A Guide to the Clinical Care of Women with HIV.* Rockville, MD: U.S. Dept. of Health and Human Services, Health Resources and Services Administration, HIV/AIDS Bureau, 2000.

Centers for Disease Control and Prevention. "Guidelines for Preventing Opportunistic Infections Among HIV-Infected Persons—2002." *Morbidity and Mortality Weekly Report* 51 (RR08) (June 14, 2002): 1–46.

———. "Guidelines for Using Antiretroviral Agents Among HIV-Infection Adults and Adolescents." *Morbidity and Mortality Weekly Report* 51 (RR07) (May 17, 2002): 1.

———. "HIV Prevention Strategic Plan through 2005." Available online at *www.cdc.gov/nchstp/od/hiv_plan/default.htm*, January 2001.

———. "Pneumocystis pneumonia—Los Angeles. 1981." *Morbidity and Mortality Weekly Report* 45(34) (August 30, 1996): 729–733.

———. "Prevention and Treatment of Tuberculosis Among Patients Infected with HIV: Principles of Therapy and Revised Recommendations." *Morbidity and Mortality Weekly Report* 47 (RR20) (October 30, 1998): 1–51.

———. "U.S. Public Health Service Task Force Recommendations for Use of Antiretroviral Drugs in Pregnant HIV-1 Infected Women for Maternal Health and Interventions To Reduce Perinatal HIV-1 Transmission in the United States." *Morbidity and Mortality Weekly Report* 51 (RR18) (November 22, 2002): 1–38.

Farmer, Paul. *Infections and Inequalities: The Modern Plagues.* Berkeley, CA: University of California Press, 1999.

"In their own words: NIH Researchers Recall the Early Years of AIDS." Available online at *http://aidshistory.nih.edu.*

Shilts, Randy. *And the Band Played on: Politics, People, and the AIDS Epidemic.* New York: St. Martin's Press, 1987.

Valdiserri, Ronald O., ed. *Dawning Answers: How the HIV/AIDS Epidemic Has Helped to Strengthen Public Health.* New York: Oxford University Press, 2003.

Further Reading

Books

Banish, Roslyn. *Focus on Living: Portraits of Americans with HIV and AIDS.* Amherst: MA: University of Massachusetts Press, 2003.

Bartlett, John G., and Joel E. Gallant. *Medical Management of HIV Infection,* 2003 Ed. Available online at *http://www.hopkins-aids.edu.*

Crawford, Dorothy H. *The Invisible Enemy: A Natural History of Viruses.* New York: Oxford University Press, 2002.

Matthews, Dawn, ed. *AIDS Sourcebook: Basic Consumer Health Information About Acquired Immune Deficiency Syndrome (AIDS) and Human Immunodeficiency Virus (HIV) Infection.* Detroit, MI: Omnigraphics, 2003.

Mayer, K.H., and H.F. Pizer, eds. *The Emergence of AIDS: The Impact on Immunology, Microbiology and Public Health.* Washington, DC: American Public Health Association, 2000.

Stine, Gerald. *AIDS Update 2003.* Upper Saddle River, NJ: Prentice Hall, 2003.

Journal Articles

Connor, E.M., R.S. Sperling, R. Gelber, et al. "Reduction of Maternal Infant Transmission of Human Immunodeficiency Virus Type 1 with Zidovudine Treatment. Pediatric AIDS Clinical Trials Group Protocol 076 Study Group." *New England Journal of Medicine* 331 (1994): 1173–1180.

Hammer, S.M., K.E. Squires, M.D. Hughes, et al. "A Controlled Trial of Two Nucleoside Analogues Plus Indinavir in Persons with Human Immunodeficiency Virus Infection and CD4 Cell Counts of 200 per Cubic Millimeter or Less." *New England Journal of Medicine* 337 (1997): 725–733.

Palella, F.J., Jr., K.M. Delaney, A.C. Moorman, et al. "Declining Morbidity and Mortality Among Patients with Advanced Human Immunodeficiency Virus Infection. HIV Outpatient Study Investigators." *New England Journal of Medicine* 338 (1998): 853–860.

Zhu, T., B.T. Korber, A.J. Nahmias, et al. "An African HIV-1 Sequence From 1959 and Implications for the Origin of the Epidemic." *Nature* 391 (1998): 594–597.

Websites

AIDS Education Global
  Information System (AEGiS)
  www.aegis.com

AIDS Info, U.S. Department of
  Health and Human Services
  www.aidsinfo.nih.gov

All the Virology on the WWW: The Big Picture Book of Viruses
  www.virolgy.net/Big Virology.BVHomePage.html

Centers for Disease
  Control and Prevention
  www.cdc.gov

Johns Hopkins AIDS Service,
  Johns Hopkins University
  www.hopkins-aids.edu

UNAIDS: The Joint United Nations
  Programme on HIV/AIDS
  www.unaids.org

United States Food and Drug Information,
  Information about HIV/AIDS
  www.fda.gov/oashi/aids/hiv.html

United States National Library of Medicine,
  Specialized Information Services,
  Information about HIV/AIDS
  http://www.sis.nlm.nih.gov/HIV/HIVMain.html

World Health Organization
  www.who.int

Index

Index

Index

Index

17:	© Roger Ressmeyer/CORBIS	51d:	© Gladden Willis, MD/Visuals Unlimited
24:	Courtesy MMWR, CDC	56:	Lambda Science Artwork
27:	Associated Press, AP	58:	Lambda Science Artwork
29:	Courtesy CDC	60:	© Dr. Dennis Kunkel/Visuals Unlimited
31:	Courtesy CDC		
36:	Courtesy UNAIDS/WHO, *AIDS Epidemic Update, 2002*	79:	Lambda Science Artwork
		84:	Lambda Science Artwork
40:	Courtesy UNAIDS/WHO, *AIDS Epidemic Update, 2002*	85:	Lambda Science Artwork
		90:	Lambda Science Artwork
45:	(top) Lambda Science Artwork	93:	Lambda Science Artwork
45:	(bottom) © Dr. Hans Gelderblom/Visuals Unlimited	96:	Lambda Science Artwork
		103:	National Library of Medicine
47:	© AFP/CORBIS	119:	© Dr. Dennis Kunkel/Visuals Unlimited
51a:	© Dr. Gary Gaugler/Visuals Unlimited		
51b:	© E. Whitney/Visuals Unlimited	130–131:	CDC
51c:	© Mike Abbey/Visuals Unlimited		

Cover: ©Michael Freeman/CORBIS

HIV/AIDS trademarks

Carraguard is a registered trademark of Population Council Inc.; Combivir is a registered trademark of Glazo Group Limited Corp.; Kaletra is a registered trademark of Abbott Laboratories Corp.; K-Y is a registered trademark of Johnson and Johnson Corporation; Trizivir is a registered trademark of Glazo Group Limited Corp.; Vaseline is a registered trademark of Chesebrough-Pond's Inc.; ZnG-Gel is a trademark of Viratech Pharmaceuticals, Inc.

About the Authors

Consuelo M. Beck-Sagué, M.D. was born in Santiago de Cuba, in Cuba, and came to live in the United States in 1961, when she was 10 years old. She went to Catholic grade school, high school, and college in Erie, Pennsylvania, and then was a Volunteer in Service to America in the South Bronx, New York City, in a drug rehabilitation center. She graduated from Temple University Medical School in Philadelphia in 1978, and completed a clinical residency in pediatrics and social medicine in 1981, and sub-specialty clinical training in infectious diseases in 2000. Dr. Beck-Sagué is board-certified in pediatrics and infectious diseases and a fellow of the American Academies of Pediatrics and Microbiology. In 1985, she joined the Centers for Disease Control and Prevention (CDC) Epidemic Intelligence Service in the Division of Sexually Transmitted Diseases. Since then, she has worked at CDC as an investigator of epidemics in hospitals and clinics, and now is a medical epidemiologist working in HIV and women's health. She has conducted more than 20 epidemic and other field investigations, and has authored or co-authored over 60 peer-reviewed journal articles, book chapters and other scientific publications on sexually transmitted diseases, including HIV/AIDS, and other infectious diseases. She plays classical piano and rock electric guitar, loves to draw and paint, and still sees patients every week. This is her first book for young adults.

Writing performed by Consuelo M. Beck-Sagué in her private capacity. No official support or endorsement by CDC is intended or should be inferred.

Caridad C. Beck is 20 years old. She attends Oberlin College in Ohio and is majoring in linguistic anthropology. She is also currently studying illustration at the Manhattan School of Art and Design. She volunteers as an HIV and reproductive health peer-counselor. During her winter terms, she has conducted research on sexually transmitted STDs and knowledge and attitudes about HIV prevention in adolescents and young adults, and has been acknowledged as a co-investigator and co-author in several CDC publications and abstracts on these subjects. She aspires to be a youth fiction writer and humorist.

The late **I. Edward Alcamo** was a Distinguished Teaching Professor of Microbiology at the State University of New York at Farmingdale. Alcamo studied biology at Iona College in New York and earned his M.S. and Ph.D. degrees in microbiology at St. John's University, also in New York. He had taught at Farmingdale for over 30 years. In 2000, Alcamo won the Carski Award for Distinguished Teaching in Microbiology, the highest honor for microbiology teachers in the United States. He was a member of the American Society for Microbiology, the National Association of Biology Teachers, and the American Medical Writers Association. Alcamo authored numerous books on the subjects of microbiology, AIDS, and DNA technology as well as the award-winning textbook *Fundamentals of Microbiology*, now in its sixth edition.